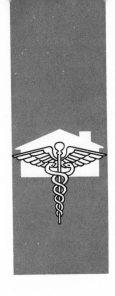

THE NEW ILLUSTRATED

MEDICAL ENCYCLOPEDIA

FOR HOME USE

VOLUME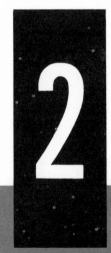

Compiled and Edited

ILLUSTRATED BY SYLVIA AND LESTER V. BERGMAN

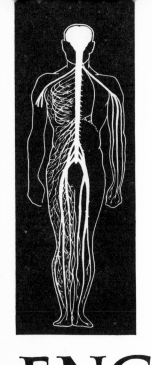

The NEW Illustrated

MEDICAL

ENCYCLOPEDIA

FOR HOME USE

A PRACTICAL GUIDE TO GOOD HEALTH

ROBERT E. ROTHENBERG, M.D., F.A.C.S.

ABRADALE PRESS *Publishers / New York*

NOTE TO THE READER

———————

The reader is advised that for disorders requiring individual examination and treatment, a doctor must be consulted, for no prescription or course of treatment is intended to be recommended in these volumes.

NEWLY REVISED EDITION

Eighth Printing, September, 1963

Library of Congress Catalog Card Number: 59-13063

———————

DESIGNED BY HOWARD MORRIS
PRINTED IN THE UNITED STATES OF AMERICA

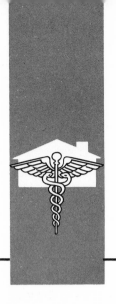

Table of Contents

This Table of Contents lists all topics in this particular volume only. For a complete Table of Contents listing all topics in the entire four volumes of this *New Illustrated Medical Encyclopedia*, see Volume One. A special section of Definitions of Common Medical Terms will be found at the end of Volume Four.

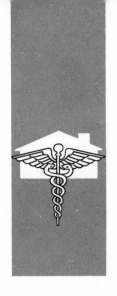

THE NEW ILLUSTRATED

MEDICAL ENCYCLOPEDIA

FOR HOME USE

20 *The Ears*

How does normal hearing take place?

Sound waves enter the external ear canal and strike the eardrum, causing it to vibrate. On the inner aspect of the drum are three tiny bones, the malleus, incus and stapes. Drum vibrations are transmitted to these bones which, in turn, vibrate and transmit the impulses to the inner ear. The inner ear is filled with a fluid surrounded by a membrane. When the stapes vibrates, the impulses are conveyed through the fluid to special nerve endings. The impulses then travel up the nerve endings to the auditory nerve, which carries them to the brain, where they are recorded as hearing.

Are there normal variations in sensitivity of hearing?

Yes. Certain individuals have a more highly developed sense of hearing than others.

How can one determine accurately how well he hears?

Accurate measurements can be taken by use of an instrument called an audiometer. Such hearing tests will show accurately the range of hearing in each ear, and thus determine sensitivity or loss.

Is it true that if a person concentrates greatly on something, he may block out sounds that are taking place within earshot?

Yes. Even though the sound waves are transmitted in the normal manner, the control of the brain is sufficiently strong so that it does not record in the conscious mind the sounds which are taking place.

Can the ears be damaged by too loud a sound or by an explosion?

Yes. Many of our young men today have deficient hearing because of explosions that took place while they served in the armed forces.

WAX (CERUMEN) IN THE EARS

Does wax occur normally in all ear canals?

Yes. It is secreted normally in all people.

What causes excessive wax in the ears?

The exact cause is unknown, but for some reason the wax-secreting glands become overactive and may produce large quantities of the substance.

What are the symptoms of excessive wax in the ears?

Sudden loss of hearing. This may occur following a bath, shower, or a swim. The wax becomes softened by the water, and as it dries it forms in such a way that it closes and obstructs the ear canal.

What is the treatment for wax in the ears?

It should be removed by a physician. It must be done carefully to prevent damage to the eardrum.

Can an individual attempt to remove the wax by himself?

Absolutely not. Great damage has been done to the ear and the eardrum by attempts to remove the wax by oneself.

Does excessive wax cause permanent damage?

No. If there is loss of hearing due to excessive wax, hearing will return immediately upon its removal.

Should people with excessive wax formation receive periodic examinations?

Yes. It is wise for them to have their physician examine their ear canals once a year.

PAIN IN THE EAR CANAL

What causes pain in the ear canal?

It is usually inflammatory in origin and may be caused by a pimple, a boil, eczema, an injury, or a foreign body which has gotten into the canal.

What is the treatment for an infection of the ear canal?

a. Warm, moist compresses.
b. If an abscess has formed, it should be incised by a physician.
c. Medications to relieve the severe pain that is usually present.

Wax in the Ears. Hearing may be diminished markedly if the external ear canal is blocked by wax. If hearing decreases, it is a good idea to visit the doctor to find out whether the ear canals contain excess wax. Such wax can be removed readily by syringing. People should *never* put things into their own ears in an attempt to clean out the wax, as serious damage may be done to the delicate hearing mechanism.

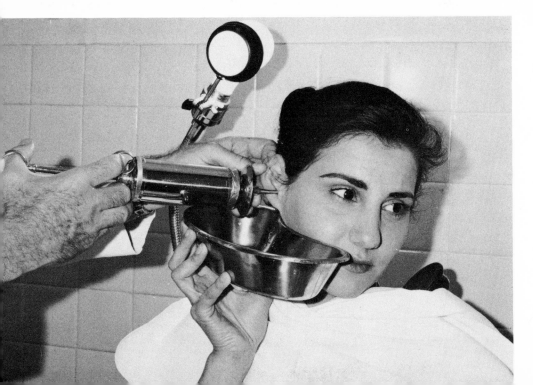

MIDDLE EAR

Where is the middle ear and what is its function?

It is on the inner side of the eardrum and connects through a narrow passageway (the Eustachian tube) with the back of the throat. It also has a direct connection with the mastoid air cells lodged in the bone behind the ear. The middle ear houses the three little bones which form a link between the eardrum and the inner ear.

What causes pain in the middle ear?

In most cases, this is due to inflammation or infection. Such inflammation is usually secondary to infection of the nose and throat. In children, recurrent attacks of earaches are indicative of enlarged adenoids.

What other conditions give rise to ear pain?

Tonsillitis, abscessed teeth, inflammation of the pharynx, sinusitis, or a tumor growth in the middle ear region.

MIDDLE EAR INFECTION
(*Otitis Media*)

What causes otitis media?

Infections of the middle ear are usually secondary to a spread, via the Eustachian tube, of an inflammation such as a cold, throat infection, inflamed adenoids. The contagious diseases of children, since they are associated with throat inflammation, also lead to middle ear and mastoid infection.

What are the symptoms of otitis media?

a. Pain in the ear.
b. Impairment of hearing.
c. Rise in temperature.
d. Examination of the eardrum will show it to be red and swollen.
e. If the eardrum has already ruptured, pus will discharge through the eardrum into the external ear canal.

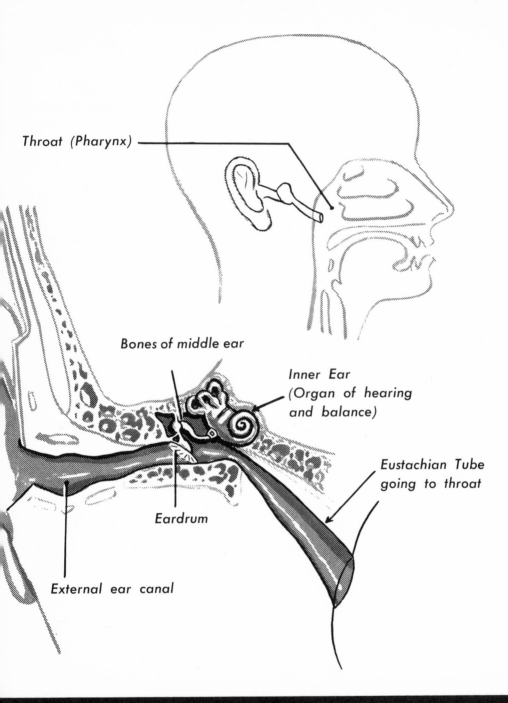

Throat (Pharynx)

Bones of middle ear

Inner Ear
(Organ of hearing
and balance)

Eustachian Tube
going to throat

Eardrum

External ear canal

Diagram of the Anatomy of the Ear. The ear is a complex mechanism, of which the external part merely acts as a receptacle for sound waves that are conducted along the ear canal. The sound waves vibrate against the eardrum and these vibrations are transmitted to the small ear bones in the middle ear. The vibrations are transmitted by these bones to the ear nerve in the inner ear which sends the impulses to the brain, where they are interpreted as sound. As seen in the accompanying diagram, the ear

Are certain families more prone to develop otitis media than others?

Yes. Owing to the particular anatomy of the Eustachian tube, certain families inherit a straighter channel. It is easier for infection to travel along the straighter channel than it is when the Eustachian tube is curved and more likely to prevent the spread of infected material.

What are the harmful results of middle ear infection?

a. Each attack results in slight thickening of the lining mucous membrane of the middle ear. Although one or even several attacks will not necessarily cause deafness, each additional inflammation leaves its mark and the end result may be loss of hearing.

b. Middle ear infections may not subside and may extend into neighboring structures to cause mastoiditis, labyrinthitis, meningitis, or brain abscess. Repeated attacks of otitis media may result in a chronic middle ear infection, with a perforated eardrum and a persistent discharge of pus from the ear canal.

What is the treatment for otitis media?

a. The best treatment is prophylactic. Children with diseased or markedly enlarged tonsils and adenoids should have them removed. People with colds should not go swimming or dive. Simple head colds should be treated and not neglected.

b. When infection of the middle ear has already taken place, adequate doses of antibiotics should be given. Nose spray or nose drops should be used to keep the nasal passages open.

c. Medications should be given to relieve the pain if it is very intense.

d. If there is a perforated drum and a discharge of pus from the ear, a specimen of the pus should be cultured and sensitivity tests performed to determine which antibiotic can be used most effectively.

When is surgery necessary in middle ear infection?

If the eardrum is bulging because of fluid in the middle ear, and the condition does not respond to the medical measures previously described, it is advisable to open the eardrums surgically. This procedure is called a myringotomy.

How is myringotomy performed?

It is done under local anesthesia in the patient's home or the physician's office. A specially devised knife is used and a small incision is made in the drum to allow the fluid or pus to escape.

How can one tell whether an infection of the middle ear has spread to involve the mastoid bone?

A mastoid infection should be suspected if:

a. There is an abrupt rise in temperature, with loss of appetite and swelling of the glands in the neck.
b. There is pain behind the ear over the mastoid bone.
c. There is tenderness on direct finger pressure over the mastoid region.
d. There is a pouching forward of the back wall of the external ear canal.
e. There is an increase in the white blood cell count.
f. There are x-ray findings which indicate involvement of the mastoid bones.
g. There is impaired hearing.
h. There may be swelling of the soft tissues behind the ear.

Are mastoid infections very common today?

No. Because of the prompt and adequate treatment of middle ear infections with the antibiotics, acute mastoiditis has become a rarity today.

What is the treatment for acute mastoiditis?

Before the advent of the sulfa drugs and the antibiotics, the wards of hospitals were filled with children suffering from mastoid infections. Today, surgery is rarely necessary for this condition. However, when a neglected case of middle ear infection does involve the mastoid bones, intensive treatment with the appropriate antibiotics will frequently clear up the infection. If this does not take place, surgery, with a scraping out of all of the infected mastoid cells, is necessary.

What may happen if a mastoid infection is permitted to go untreated?

a. Paralysis of the facial nerve may take place.

b. A bloodstream infection may take place.

c. Infection may extend into the skull and cause a meningitis or brain abscess.

d. A fatality may ultimately result if the condition goes untreated.

How is a simple mastoidectomy performed?

It may be done either through the ear canal (endaural) or by the postauricular route. In the former, an incision is made within the ear canal extending from the drum outward. In the latter approach, an incision is made behind the ear. In both instances, the infected bone is chipped and scraped away until all of the cells are uncovered and found to be healthy.

What type of anesthesia is used for mastoidectomy?

General anesthesia.

Is mastoidectomy a dangerous operation?

No.

Is hearing affected by a mastoid operation?

a. Simple mastoidectomy does not impair hearing.

b. Radical mastoidectomy for a chronic ear infection does cause loss of hearing in that ear.

What is the difference between simple and radical mastoidectomy?

A simple mastoidectomy involves removal of the mastoid air cells only. Radical mastoidectomy involves not only the removal of the mastoid cells, but also the removal of the eardrum and contents of the middle ear.

How long does it take to perform a simple mastoidectomy?

Approximately one hour.

Does the ear continue to drain pus even after a mastoidectomy?

Yes, for several days to several weeks.

Are special preoperative or postoperative medications given after mastoidectomy?

Yes. Large doses of antibiotics are utilized to control and prevent spread of infection.

How long a hospital stay is needed for mastoidectomy?

Seven to ten days.

Will it be necessary to treat the patient for a long period of time after mastoidectomy?

Yes, for several weeks.

Is the scar of mastoidectomy disfiguring?

No.

Does mastoid infection often recur after surgery?

No.

Does mastoidectomy carry with it a high mortality?

No. It is not a dangerous operation.

DEAFNESS

What causes deafness?

Impairment of hearing may be caused by any interference with the reception or transmission of sound waves along the canal through the middle ear to the inner ear and then along the auditory nerve to the brain.

When there is deafness of one ear, will the other ear become involved too?

Deafness may occasionally be limited to one ear when it is secondary to an infection, but this is not the general rule. In most cases, when one ear is involved, the other ear will show a loss of hearing sooner or later.

Do both ears tend to go deaf at the same time?

Not necessarily. There may be a wide interval, or there may be no impairment of hearing in the other ear if one ear is affected.

What kinds of deafness are encountered?

  a. Congenital deafness.
  b. Central deafness due to involvement of the brain.
  c. Perceptive deafness due to involvement of the internal ear or auditory nerve.
  d. Conductive deafness due to involvement of the middle ear or auditory canal.

What is congenital deafness?

This is a type with which one is born and is based upon the abnormal development or lack of development of the nerve of hearing.

Audiometer. Hearing can be tested accurately by an instrument known as an audiometer. This simple test is performed by placing earphones over the ears and recording the patient's ability to hear the sounds transmitted by the audiometer.

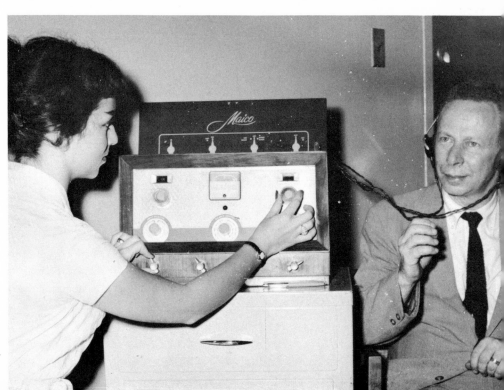

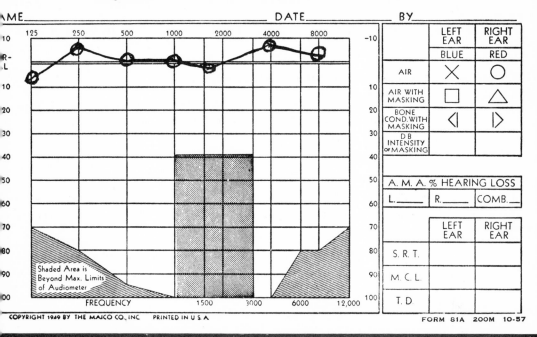

Audiogram. The audiogram is a graphic summary of the measurements of hearing loss. The particular audiogram shown here demonstrates that the patient has normal hearing.

What causes congenital deafness?

It is thought that many cases are caused by diseases which the pregnant woman has during the first few weeks of the pregnancy. Toxins from certain diseases, such as German measles, are transmitted to the young embryo and cause maldevelopment of certain organs.

What happens if a child is born deaf?

The deaf child cannot hear; therefore, he cannot imitate and thus learn to talk. These children become the deaf-mutes we see so often. In other words, the deaf-mute *could* talk if he had been able to hear and imitate the sounds of speech. There is nothing wrong with the speech mechanism of the deaf-mute.

What are the causes of inner ear deafness?

a. Diseases such as mumps, influenza, scarlet fever, and malaria.

b. Drugs such as quinine and salicylates.

c. Occupations such as boilermaking, piloting an airplane, etc.

d. Fractures through the temporal bone of the skull which traverse the ear mechanism.

e. Allergic reactions involving the labyrinth.

e. Hemorrhage into the inner ear.

f. Tumors of the nerve of hearing (the acoustic nerve).

How can deafness caused by a defect in the inner ear be distinguished from deafness caused by trouble in the middle ear?

Middle ear deafness does not involve disease of the transmission mechanism. Thus, if a vibrating tuning fork is held against the mastoid bone behind the ear, the vibrating sound is intensified as it can be transmitted through the undamaged inner ear. If the deafness is a result of disturbance in the inner ear or in the acoustic nerve, the tuning fork vibrations will not be heard.

Can deafness be helped medically?

a. If the deafness was caused by disease, such as mumps, etc., nothing can be done to improve the hearing, except by the use of hearing aids.

b. If the deafness was caused by drugs, and the use of the drug is stopped before permanent damage has occurred, hearing will improve by itself.

c. When deafness has been caused by exposure to loud noises or explosions, improvement will take place over a period of time if the patient is removed from such noises.

d. Deafness following fracture of the temporal bone or hemorrhage may recede as time passes, but little can be done medically to influence this change.

e. Deafness due to tumors of the acoustic nerve can be improved by surgical removal of the tumor.

What causes middle ear (conductive) deafness?

a. Impacted wax.

b. A foreign body in the external ear canal.

c. A discharge in the canal.

d. Narrowing of the canal due to inflammation of the skin of the canal.

e. Tumors of the external auditory canal.

f. Perforated eardrums.

g. Inflammation of the middle ear.

h. Tumor of the middle ear.

i. Lack of mobility of the stapes bone in the middle ear.

j. A blocked Eustachian tube.

What is the incidence of conduction deafness?

It is estimated that about five out of every hundred people have deafness caused by disturbance in their conduction apparatus. Fortunately, only one of these five people has impairment to such degree that it requires medical attention.

What are some of the medical measures used to improve conduction deafness?

If deafness has been due to wax in the external ear, to a foreign body in the canal, to an inflammation in the canal, to a middle ear infection, or to a blocked Eustachian tube, this can be helped readily by medical management by the nose and throat specialist. If, however, maximum benefit has been obtained from medical measures and impairment still exists, people with conductive deafness should use hearing aids.

Are hearing aids effective?

Yes. There are wonderful new hearing aids being manufactured and constant improvements are being made all the time.

Is x-ray therapy or radium ever used for the treatment of deafness?

In certain cases where the Eustachian tube is blocked by an overgrowth of lymphoid tissue, especially in children, x-ray or radium treatment may cause this tissue to shrink and thus improve hearing.

Is surgery helpful in the treatment of deafness?

Yes, in certain types of deafness. If the deafness is caused by the presence of fluid in the middle ear, an incision in the eardrum which permits the fluid to escape will often be followed by a complete return of hearing.

In cases of otosclerosis, a form of conductive deafness, there are operative procedures which may prove beneficial.

What is otosclerosis?

Otosclerosis is a disease of the inner ear.

What are the harmful results of otosclerosis?

Otosclerosis is the most common cause of deafness, usually of the conductive type.

Does otosclerosis always cause deafness?

No.

What are the symptoms of otosclerosis?

Deafness is the outstanding symptom, but occasionally it causes noises in the ears. There are no abnormal ear findings on examination.

What is the treatment for otosclerosis?

There is no known cure for this condition. In many cases, the deafness can be lessened greatly either by the fenestration operation or by mobilization of the stapes.

What is the fenestration operation?

One in which a new opening is made in the bone overlying the inner ear. The eardrum is then placed over this new opening so as to transmit sound waves through it.

Which deaf people can be helped by the fenestration operation?

Those whose deafness is caused by rigidity of the stapes bone of the middle ear. This operation is performed only if the auditory nerve functions normally. Also, the eardrum must be normal.

At what age can the fenestration operation be performed?

There are no age limits. Children can be operated upon, if indicated.

Is the fenestration operation painful?

No.

What anesthesia is used for the fenestration operation?

Local anesthesia.

Is there a noticeable scar from the fenestration operation?

No, the incisions are made within the ear canal.

Are both ears operated upon at the same time in the fenestration operation?

No; they are done separately.

Are skin grafts ever used to close the wound in the ear canal when performing the fenestration operation?

Yes. This is done in most cases. A small piece of skin is obtained from the patient's own thigh.

What are the complications of the fenestration operation?

There are not many and they do not occur too often. However, when they do occur they take the form of dizziness, noises in the ear, or, more rarely, infection with discharge from the ear.

How long a hospital stay is necessary after a fenestration operation?

Five to nine days.

How soon can one return to work after the fenestration operation?

Within three to four weeks, when the dizziness has abated.

What percentage of those patients who undergo the fenestration operation are benefited?

Seventy to 80 per cent.

Are the benefits of surgery permanent?

Yes, in the great majority of cases.

Can a patient be reoperated upon if the fenestration operation was not successful?

Yes.

When should the operation with mobilization of the stapes be used rather than the fenestration operation?

Since the mobilization operation is a simpler procedure than the fenestration operation, and, when successful, gives a greater return of the hearing function, it should be tried before the fenestration operation is attempted.

If the mobilization of the stapes operation is unsuccessful, the fenestration operation can then be done.

What is meant by mobilization of the stapes?

In otosclerosis, the stapes bone is rigid and fixed and is therefore unable to transmit the sound waves from the eardrum to the fluid of the inner ear. In this operation, the eardrum is lifted from its normal position, thus exposing the stapes. A fine instrument is then used to manipulate this tiny bone so as to free it from its adhesions or restrictions. The eardrum is then placed back into its original position.

What anesthesia is used for the mobilization operation?
Local anesthesia.

Is there a visible scar from mobilization of the stapes?
No.

Are skin grafts necessary for mobilization of the stapes operation?
No.

What are possible complications of the mobilization operation?

a. Infection, with discharge of pus from the ear.
b. Failure to obtain improved hearing.

How long a hospital stay is necessary after a mobilization of the stapes procedure?

One to two days.

Are the results from mobilization operations permanent?

Since this operation is a relatively new one, this question cannot be answered at this time. However, there are patients who still have improved hearing as long as five years after surgery.

If mobilization of the stapes fails, can the operation be done over?

Yes, but occasionally the stapes bone is damaged during the performance of the operation. In that event, the fenestration operation can be attempted with a reasonable chance of success.

EQUILIBRIUM

What is equilibrium?

It is the inner consciousness of, and the maintenance of, the normal posture and balance of the individual in standing, walking, and carrying out normal physical activity.

On what does equilibrium depend?

It depends on three interrelated factors:
a. The eyes.
b. The skin and muscle-position sense.
c. The vestibular labyrinth mechanism of the inner ear and its connections to the brain.

Must all three of these above factors be working perfectly in order to maintain equilibrium?

No. Balance can be maintained if two of the above three factors function properly.

What is meant by vertigo?

Vertigo is a sensation of disturbed position, posture, or balance. In other words, it is an abnormality of the equilibrium. It is a symptom and not a disease.

ACOUSTIC NERVE TUMORS

Are acoustic nerve tumors common, and what is the treatment for them?

Acoustic nerve tumors are rather common and must be treated by the neurosurgeon.

What are the symptoms of an acoustic nerve tumor?

a. Vertigo and dizziness.
b. Buzzing, hissing, and ringing in the ear on the involved side.
c. Impairment of hearing.
d. Weakness or paralysis of the facial muscles.
e. Pain on the involved side of the face.
f. Headache.

MENIÈRE'S SYNDROME

What is Menière's syndrome?

It is a disease characterized by sudden attacks of vertigo, buzzing or ringing in the ears, impairment of hearing, with occasional episodes of headache and vomiting.

What causes the Menière's syndrome?

The cause is not known.

What is the treatment for Menière's syndrome?

The restriction of sodium from the diet and the use of nicotinic acid have proved helpful in some cases. When the disease has become so severe that it incapacitates the patient, surgery is sometimes advised to sever the vestibular part of the acoustic nerve. Unfortunately, this surgical procedure may also destroy hearing.

PLASTIC SURGERY OF THE EAR

For what conditions is plastic surgery of the ear recommended?

a. Protruding ears.
b. Folded or lop ears.
c. Deformities of the external ear.
d. Deformities of the external ear canal.

What is the usual cause of these conditions?

They are deformities of the ear cartilage present since birth.

Does the shape of the ear tend to run in families or be inherited?
Yes.

Will an infant develop deformed ears because he lies upon them when they are in a folded position?
No. This is a common misconception.

Are folded and lop ears seen on one side only?
Yes, but there are many cases in which both ears are misshapen.

Is hearing disturbed by deformities of the external ear?
No.

Will plastic surgery upon the external ear influence hearing?
No.

Can large ears be made smaller?
Yes, through plastic surgery.

Is plastic surgery upon the ears difficult?
No. The only difficult case is when the external ear is totally or partially lacking. In such an instance, very complicated skin grafting is required to create a new external ear.

At what age should a child be operated upon for correction of deformed ears?
When the child is old enough to cooperate and not disturb his bandages. This means usually just before school age, between the ages of four and six. Some surgeons advocate not operating upon these children until they reach the age of thirteen or fourteen.

What operative procedure is carried out for protruding or lop ears?
An elliptical skin incision is made behind the ear and an elliptical section of skin and cartilage is removed. The skin edges are then sutured one to the other, which brings the ear back into normal position and appearance. A firm dressing is applied so that the ear will remain in its new position, the head is snugly bandaged, and

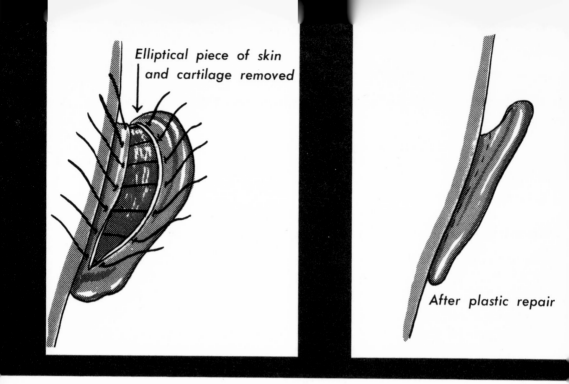

Elliptical piece of skin
and cartilage removed

After plastic repair

Lop Ears. This diagram shows how plastic repair of lop ears is carried out. It is a simple operation with excellent results. Children may become very self-conscious because of folded or lop ears, and it is unnecessary for them to go through life with such a deformity.

the bandages are left in place for about ten days, until solid healing has taken place.

Is there swelling of the ear following these operations?

Yes, but this will disappear within a few days to several weeks.

Are the cosmetic results of these operations good?

Yes. In the great majority of cases they are excellent.

What anesthesia is used for operations of this type?

For children, general anesthesia. For adults, local anesthesia.

Are the scars of these operations visible?

No, as the incisions are behind the ears in the folds of the skin lines.

How long a period of hospitalization is necessary?

From two to five days.

If the results are not perfectly satisfactory, can these operations be redone?

Yes. Reoperation may correct any residual deformity.

CONGENITAL DEFORMITIES OF THE EAR

What are the birth deformities of the ear?

These abnormalities are very rare. There are two usual forms:

a. Absence of the external ear canal. This is usually accompanied by maldevelopment of the middle ear, although the inner ear which controls the sense of balance is usually intact.

b. Absence of the external ear. In these cases, if there is a normally developed external ear canal, middle ear, and inner ear, hearing is not greatly interfered with.

How common are these congenital deformities of the ear?

Absence of the external ear canal occurs in approximately one in two thousand cases of ear disease. Absence of the whole external ear is quite rare, but one does see partial deformities in the formation of the external ear. Both of these deformities are more likely to occur on one side than on both sides.

Can surgery be helpful for congenital deformities of the ear?

To construct an external ear canal in these cases is usually not of great value, since hearing cannot be restored. This is due to the fact that the eardrum and the middle ear are usually underdeveloped. There are extensive plastic operations for the construction of a new external ear; these operations may be worth while psychologically, but the ultimate results are not too acceptable from a cosmetic point of view.

21

The Esophagus

What is the esophagus?

It is a muscular tube which connects the pharynx, or back of the throat, to the stomach. Through it, swallowed food and fluid are conducted to the stomach. The esophagus has no digestive function, but acts merely as a conduit.

Is the drinking of excessively hot liquids harmful to the esophagus?

Yes, as it may burn the lining membrane. Also, some investigators believe that the taking of extremely hot foods, over a period of many years, may stimulate cancer formation.

Is the drinking of excessively cold liquids harmful to the esophagus?

No.

Can one choke from swallowing too large a quantity of food at one time?

If food enters the esophagus and not the trachea (windpipe), choking does not take place. However, taking too much food in one swallow may cause it to become stuck somewhere along the course of the esophagus. This may require the passage of an esophagoscope in order to remove the excess food particles.

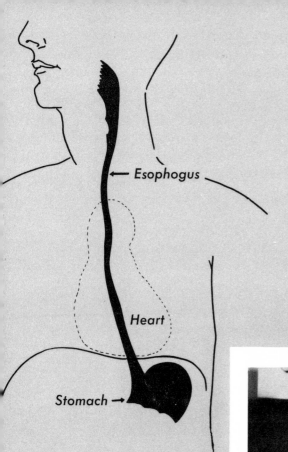

Esophagus. The diagram shows the normal esophagus as it traverses the chest cavity and empties into the stomach below the diaphragm.

X-ray of Esophagus. This x-ray shows the normal esophagus within the chest cavity. It should be noted that its contours are smooth and that no constrictions obstruct the passage of the barium.

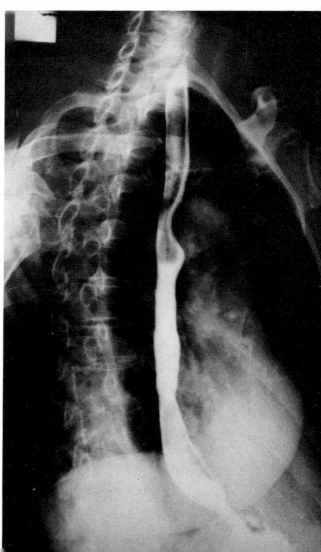

What is the significance of inability to swallow?

It usually signifies an obstruction due either to a mechanical cause or to spasm.

What does it mean if there is regurgitation of undigested food?

It signifies either an obstruction of the esophagus or the presence of an esophageal diverticulum (pouch).

What is the significance of regurgitation of sour-tasting food or stomach contents?

This is caused in most instances by conditions within the stomach, duodenum, or gall bladder, and not by esophageal disease.

What is the significance of tightness in the throat, especially in women in their forties?

This is a hysterical tightening of the muscles of the throat encountered in women during their menopausal years. It is not due to organic disease and does not involve the esophagus.

What are some of the common conditions affecting the esophagus?

a. Birth deformities.
b. Inflammatory conditions.
c. Injuries, including burns and foreign bodies.
d. Diverticulum of the esophagus.
e. Chronic spasm (achalasia).
f. Varicose veins.
g. Tumors.

BIRTH DEFORMITIES

What types of birth deformities of the esophagus are encountered?

The most common type of birth deformity is known as a tracheo-esophageal fistula. This is an abnormal communication between the esophagus and the trachea (windpipe). As a result of such an abnormal opening, saliva, milk, or other swallowed materials get into the lungs and cause irritation, often resulting in pneumonia.

Is tracheo-esophageal fistula a serious condition?

Yes. If untreated, it always results in death.

What is the proper treatment for these fistulae?

Surgery must be performed promptly. This will involve severing the abnormal communication and stitching the openings left in the esophagus and trachea.

What are the chances for recovery following this operation?

The mortality is approximately 35 per cent. However, formerly, in the days before operation was feasible in this type of case, the mortality was 100 per cent.

Are there other birth deformities of the esophagus?

Yes. There may be an interruption in the continuity of the esophagus, with failure of the structure to reach the stomach. This is known as congenital atresia. Occasionally, a web, or diaphragm, is found coursing across the passageway. Such an abnormality may completely obstruct the channel of the esophagus.

What is the treatment for an incompletely developed esophagus?

By an extremely extensive operation, performed through the chest, the two normal ends of the esophagus are sutured together. If the lower half of the esophagus is not developed at all, it may be necessary to bring the stomach up into the chest and sew it to the lowermost portion of normally developed section of the esophagus.

Is there any urgency in the performance of this operation?

Yes. This operation must be performed as soon as the diagnosis of the congenital abnormality is made. If surgery is not.instituted immediately, the condition will result in death of the child.

What procedure is carried out for a congenital web of the esophagus?

It must be removed surgically. This is not as serious an operation as for congenital atresia.

INFLAMMATION OF THE ESOPHAGUS
(Esophagitis)

What conditions cause inflammation of the esophagus?

Inflammation of the esophagus (esophagitis) is found in association either with a hernia of the diaphragm (hiatus hernia) or with an ulcer in the stomach. In hiatus hernia, a portion of the stomach protrudes into the chest cavity through a widening of the opening in the diaphragm. This permits stomach contents and juices to go up into the esophagus, where they often cause irritation and set up a secondary inflammatory reaction. Patients with ulcers in the duodenum are also prone to regurgitate highly acid contents from the stomach into the lower portion of the esophagus. This may create an esophagitis.

Is esophagitis a serious condition?

Yes. It is serious because it can result in a rupture of the esophagus, bleeding, or stricture formation, with consequent interference with swallowing.

What is the proper treatment for esophagitis?

The underlying cause must be removed. If a hiatus hernia is present, it should be corrected by surgery. If a duodenal ulcer is present, adequate medical treatment should be instituted. This should include a bland diet, drugs which prevent spasm, and medicines which counteract the excess acid secretions of the stomach.

Is it ever necessary surgically to remove that portion of the esophagus affected by esophagitis?

If the esophagitis fails to respond to the usual medical measures, its removal, followed by re-establishment of the continuity of the esophagus, may be necessary to bring about a cure.

Is removal of a portion of the esophagus a serious operation?

Yes, indeed; but approximately 90 per cent will recover.

INJURIES OF THE ESOPHAGUS

What are some of the common injuries to the esophagus?

The most frequent injury to the esophagus is caused by the swallowing of corrosives, such as lye. All too often this happens to small children because adults have carelessly failed to keep these dangerous substances out of a child's reach.

What changes occur in the esophagus as a result of swallowing corrosive substances?

Severe esophagitis, complicated by stricture formation, may result from swallowing lye.

What is the treatment for this kind of injury?

The esophagitis is treated much the same as esophagitis from any other condition. If a stricture develops, it is treated by forceful, frequent dilatations over a period of several months. If dilatations do not produce a satisfactory increase in the diameter of the passageway, then removal of the constricted portion of esophagus may be required. If the involved area is extensive, it may be necessary to bring the stomach up into the chest and to suture it to that portion of esophagus which is normal and uninvolved in stricture formation.

What other types of injury of the esophagus are encountered?

The esophagus is, on rare occasions, ruptured as a result of severe vomiting. It may also be perforated by the swallowing of a sharp foreign body such as a safety pin, a fish bone, or a denture.

What is the management for a ruptured esophagus?

Rupture of the esophagus demands immediate surgery with closure of the opening and drainage of the chest cavity. On occasion, if the patient's condition is too poor to permit surgery, this condition may be treated conservatively by surgical drainage of the chest. In such cases, a permanent leak from the esophagus may develop, which will eventually require surgical correction.

385

DIVERTICULUM OF THE ESOPHAGUS

What is a diverticulum of the esophagus?

It is an outpouching, or hernia, of the mucous membrane through the muscle wall of the esophagus, which produces a sac-like protrusion in an otherwise smooth mucous membrane channel.

Where are diverticula usually located?

The most common location is in that portion of the esophagus which traverses the neck. They may also be located within the chest, in the mid-portion of the esophagus, or in the lowermost portion, near the diaphragm.

Do diverticula ordinarily produce symptoms?

Those in the neck usually cause symptoms because they tend to fill with fluid and grow larger, thus leading to obstruction of the esophagus. In addition, fluid or food which collects within the diverticulum may be ejected into the main passageway of the esophagus, thus causing regurgitation or vomiting. Occasionally, bleeding takes place from a diverticulum, and, in rare instances, malignancy may develop within one of these sacs.

Do all diverticula cause symptoms?

No. Only those that occur in the neck or in the lowermost portion of the esophagus are symptomatic. Those that occur within the mid-portion of the esophagus ordinarily do not cause symptoms, but they often do lead to inflammation of lymph glands within the chest cavity.

What treatment is recommended for diverticula of the esophagus?

Surgical removal of those diverticula which cause symptoms. If the diverticulum is located in the neck, the incision is made in the neck. If the diverticulum is located in the lowermost portion of the esophagus, the operation is performed through the chest cavity.

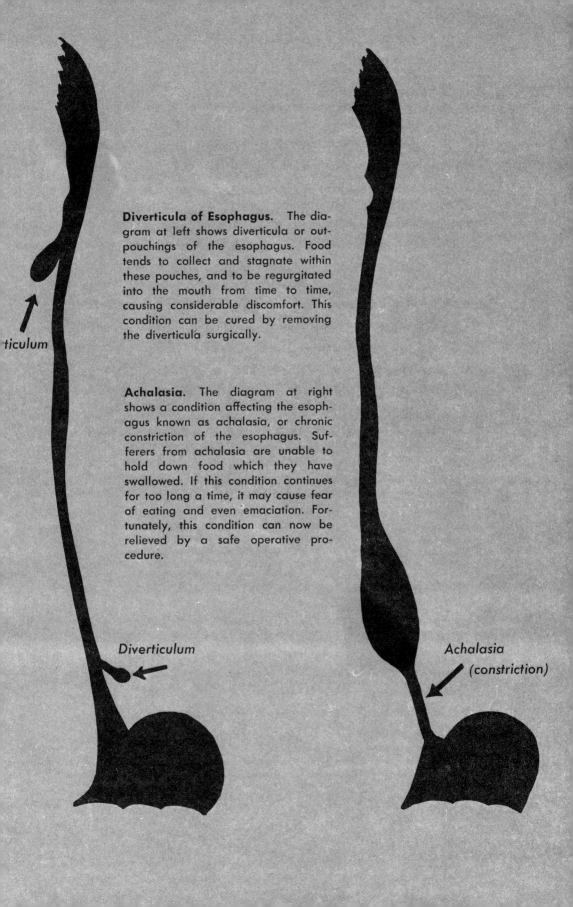

Diverticula of Esophagus. The diagram at left shows diverticula or outpouchings of the esophagus. Food tends to collect and stagnate within these pouches, and to be regurgitated into the mouth from time to time, causing considerable discomfort. This condition can be cured by removing the diverticula surgically.

Achalasia. The diagram at right shows a condition affecting the esophagus known as achalasia, or chronic constriction of the esophagus. Sufferers from achalasia are unable to hold down food which they have swallowed. If this condition continues for too long a time, it may cause fear of eating and even emaciation. Fortunately, this condition can now be relieved by a safe operative procedure.

ticulum

Diverticulum

Achalasia
(constriction)

ACHALASIA
(*Esophageal Spasm*)

What is achalasia, or spasm of the esophagus?

This is a condition in which certain nerves of the esophagus are absent, probably since birth. As a result of this deficiency, there is inability of the lower end of the esophagus to dilate and relax. As a consequence of this continued spasm, the esophagus above the area of spasm becomes tremendously widened and dilated.

What causes achalasia?

It is thought to be associated with a birth deformity in which there is absence of certain nerve elements within the wall of the esophagus.

What age groups are usually affected by this disease?

People in their twenties and thirties.

What symptoms are associated with achalasia?

The most common complaint is inability to swallow normally. This symptom becomes progressive and severe. In addition, there is often a foul odor to the breath because of retained food particles within the esophagus. Sufferers from this condition are undernourished and show evidences of marked weight loss.

What is the treatment for achalasia?

Seventy-five per cent of patients with achalasia will respond satisfactorily to repeated dilatations of the esophagus. However, about 25 per cent will require operation because they fail to obtain relief from repeated dilatations.

What type of operation is performed for achalasia?

The thickened muscle fibers overlying the area of spasm are severed in a longitudinal direction. This permits outpouching of the mucous membrane of the esophagus at that site and creates an inability of the esophageal muscles to contract or become spastic.

Is this a safe operative procedure?

Yes. It is carried out through an incision in the chest but is not associated with great surgical risk.

What are the results of this operation?

The majority of patients are greatly improved, but an occasional patient may develop esophagitis as a complication.

VARICOSE VEINS OF THE ESOPHAGUS

What causes varicose veins of the esophagus?

Obstruction of the portal circulation, that is, the circulation of blood through the liver. This is seen in cirrhosis. (See Chapter 36, on the Liver.) Since the blood cannot get from the intestinal tract through the liver, it by-passes that organ and travels along the veins of the esophagus. This vastly increased blood volume causes the esophageal veins to dilate and become varicosed.

What harm can result from esophageal varicosities?

Eventually, when the veins become too distended and dilated, they may rupture and cause a tremendous hemorrhage.

How is the diagnosis of esophageal varicosities made?

a. By noting the evidences of cirrhosis of the liver.
b. By x-ray studies of the esophagus after taking a barium swallow.
c. By noting the bringing up of large quantities of blood through the mouth.

What can be done to relieve esophageal varicosities?

a. Attempts should be made to relieve the portal circulatory obstruction. This is attempted either by suturing the large portal vein (in the abdomen) to the vena cava, or by suturing the main vein of the spleen to the main vein of the left kidney.
b. When life-threatening hemorrhage from esophageal varicosities is taking place, it may be necessary to open the chest, isolate and open the esophagus, and tie off the bleeding veins.

389

TUMORS OF THE ESOPHAGUS

What are the different types of tumors of the esophagus?

    a. Benign tumors.   b. Malignant tumors.

What is the relative frequency of tumors of the esophagus?

It is said that approximately 1 per cent of all deaths from cancer are due to cancer of the esophagus. Benign tumors occur much less frequently.

Is there any variation in the incidence of this disease in either sex?

Yes. Males are much more commonly affected than females.

What are the usual age ranges for cancer of the esophagus?

Fifty to seventy years.

What symptoms are associated with malignancies of the esophagus?

    a. Difficulty in swallowing
    b. Loss of desire to eat
    c. Weakness and weight loss

What is the treatment for cancer of the esophagus?

Either surgery or x-ray therapy, or a combination of both.

How effective are these forms of treatment in the cure of the disease?

Radiation treatment rarely results in a cure for a cancer of the esophagus. Surgery can affect a cure in approximately 20 per cent of all patients with cancer involving the lowermost portion of the esophagus.

Are benign tumors of the esophagus curable?

Yes. Practically all patients with this condition can be cured by surgical excision of the tumor.

What type of operation is performed for malignant esophageal tumors?

Those that can be attacked most successfully are usually located in the middle or lower third of the esophagus. In these cases, through a chest incision, it is possible to remove that part of the esophagus involved in tumor formation and a generous portion of normal esophagus surrounding it. Through an opening made in the diaphragm, the stomach is drawn up into the chest and is sutured to the remaining stump of esophagus.

What other forms of operation are available for cancer of the esophagus?

In another, less commonly used operation, the tumor and adjacent esophagus are widely removed and replaced by a plastic tube. This has a disadvantage, however, of being followed in many cases by leakage.

Are operations for removal of esophageal malignancy serious?

Yes. It is one of the most formidable of all operations and should be performed only by a specially trained surgeon.

22 *The Eyes*

Is it necessary for an eye specialist to perform an eye examination, or is an optometrist capable of performing the entire examination?

When an optometrist works in association with an ophthalmologist, it is often sufficient to have him examine the eyes if it is solely for the purpose of obtaining eyeglasses. However, an examination by an ophthalmologist (eye specialist) is always advisable when the patient feels something is wrong with his eyes.

How often should one have a routine checkup of the eyes?

The average person should have his eyes checked at least every two years.

The nearsighted patient should be checked every six to twelve months.

The farsighted patient under the age of forty should be examined at least every two years.

All people over the age of forty should be checked every year.

What are the common causes of eyestrain?

a. The need for eyeglasses.

b. Reading under a poor light.

c. Reading in any position other than sitting up.

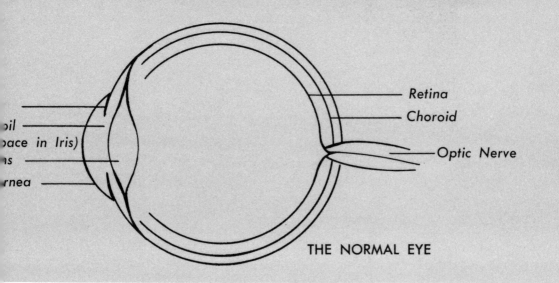

oil
ace in Iris)
s
rnea

Retina
Choroid
Optic Nerve

THE NORMAL EYE

The Normal Eye. This diagram illustrates the mechanism of sight. Light rays pass through the pupil and through the lens, where they are bent so that they focus on the retina in the rear of the eye. This apparatus is almost exactly like a camera, with the pupil corresponding to the opening of the camera. The lens of the eye is similar to the lens of the camera and the retina in the back of the eye is comparable to the photographic film in a camera.

Testing the Eyes for Glasses (Refraction). People should have their eyes tested about once a year, as changes in vision tend to take place as one ages. Changes in eyeglass prescriptions are sometimes difficult to adjust to, but it is always wise to use the glasses your oculist recommends.

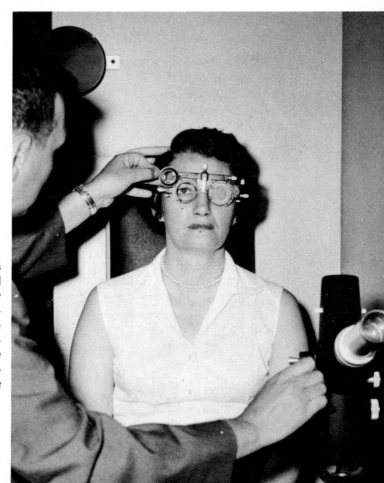

What are the symptoms of eyestrain?

Blurring of vision, smarting and burning of the eyes, slight tearing, and headaches.

Can eyestrain be caused by reading too much?

Yes.

What is the treatment for eyestrain?

a. Wearing corrective glasses.
b. Reading under a good light.
c. Sitting in a good reading position.
d. Proper rest periods.
e. Eye drops, prescribed by a physician to reduce eyestrain.

Can permanent damage to the eye result from overuse?

No. The eyes will recover if properly treated.

Why do people have different colored eyes?

The color of the eyes depends on the amount of pigment in the iris. The less pigment there is, the bluer the eye; the more pigment, the browner the eye.

Is it significant if a person has one eye of a different color from the other?

No. This has no significance whatever.

Is it natural for the pupils of children's eyes to be exceptionally large?

Yes. As a child grows older, the pupil will appear smaller.

What causes tearing of the eyes?

This may be due to irritation from excessively bright lights, a sharp wind, smoke, inflammation of the eye, a foreign body in the eye, or a blocked tear duct. It occurs more frequently in older people.

What are the common causes for itching and swelling of the eyes and lids?

Itching may be due to an allergic condition, such as hay fever or sensitivity to smoke or face powder or soap.

Swelling of the lids should be a signal to see your physician to make sure that your kidney function is normal.

Slight swelling of the lids is sometimes caused by insufficient sleep.

What causes red lid margins?

This condition may be caused by exposure to irritating smoke, dust, or wind, eyestrain, allergy, or chronic conjunctivitis. Children may develop red lid margins when they rub their eyes with dirty hands.

What causes the spots that are seen floating in front of the eyes?

Spots are caused by opacities of protein matter which float in the back portion (vitreous) of the eyeball. These opacities become visible as small spots or threads and are usually seen when a person looks at a bright background such as a clear sky or white paper. Usually, they are of no significance unless associated with blurring of vision. If vision is blurred, see your eye doctor for a thorough examination.

What causes bulging of the eyes?

Bulging or prominent eyes may be due to overactivity of the thyroid gland, or to excessive nearsightedness. In some people it is a normal anatomical feature and has no significance.

How does one treat the so-called "black eye"?

For the first twenty-four hours, cold wet compresses should be applied to lessen swelling. After twenty-four hours, warm compresses should be used to hasten absorption of the blood clot.

NEARSIGHTEDNESS
(Myopia)

What is nearsightedness?

In nearsightedness, the eyeball is longer than it should normally be for that individual. Vision is better for near objects than for distant objects.

395

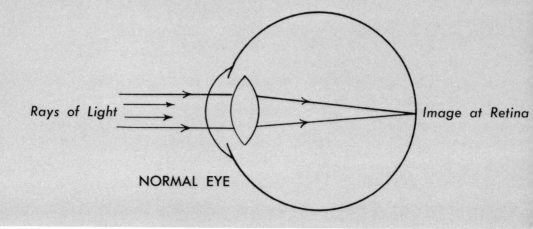

Rays of Light

Image at Retina

NORMAL EYE

The Normal Eye.   This diagram shows another view of the normal eye, with the light rays focusing exactly upon the retina in the back of the eye. When these rays hit the retina they are transmitted to the brain along nerve pathways and are interpreted by the brain as sight.

How common is nearsightedness?

About one-third of all people who wear glasses are nearsighted.

Are boys more likely to be nearsighted than girls?

No.

Is nearsightedness inherited?

It sometimes does appear to run in families, particularly if both parents are nearsighted.

Can anything be done to prevent nearsightedness?

No.

Nearsighted Eye (Myopia).   The diagram of the nearsighted eye shows the image focusing in front of the retina. When this defect is corrected by eyeglasses, the image is made to focus exactly upon the retina.

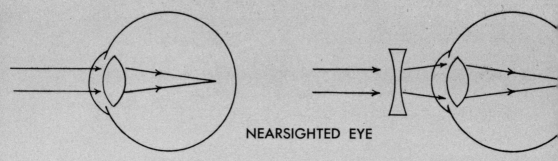

NEARSIGHTED EYE

(Image focused in front of Retina)

Corrected by Lens (eyeglasses)

Does nearsightedness tend to get better by itself?

No.

Will wearing the proper eyeglasses lead to an improvement in near-sightedness?

Yes.

Is it ever bad to wear eyeglasses for nearsightedness?

No.

How early can children be fitted for eyeglasses for nearsightedness?

Usually at three years, but, if necessary, at one year of age.

How can the doctor detect nearsightedness in small children?

By shining a light in the eye and performing a test known as retinoscopy.

Why does nearsightedness get worse as one matures?

As the body grows, the eyeball gets larger.

Should nearsighted people spare their eyes from excess reading?

No. This is necessary only if the nearsightedness is very severe.

Does watching television have any adverse effect on the eyes of near-sighted people?

None at all.

What are contact lenses?

These are molded plastic lenses which fit directly over the eyeballs and therefore disguise the fact that glasses are being worn.

When are contact lenses recommended in nearsightedness?

When the nearsightedness is of moderate severity and the patient does not want to give the appearance of wearing glasses.

Are contact lenses worn directly against the eyeball harmful to the eyes?

Not if they are well fitted.

Is there any medication to help nearsightedness?

No.

Is there any surgical procedure which can help nearsightedness?

In extreme cases of nearsightedness, removal of the lens of the eye may help to decrease nearsightedness.

Does nearsightedness ever lead to blindness?

In the very rare case, nearsightedness may lead to detachment of the retina, with some loss of vision. (See the section on Detached Retina in this chapter.)

FARSIGHTEDNESS
(Presbyopia)

What is farsightedness?

In farsightedness, the eyeball is shorter than it should normally be for that individual. Vision is better for distant than for near objects. In marked cases, vision is also blurred for distant objects.

How common is farsightedness?

About one-third of all people who wear glasses are farsighted.

Are boys more likely to be farsighted than girls?

No.

Is farsightedness inherited, or does it tend to run in families?

No.

Can anything be done to prevent farsightedness?

No.

Does farsightedness tend to get better by itself?

No, but in growing children, farsightedness may change into near-sightedness.

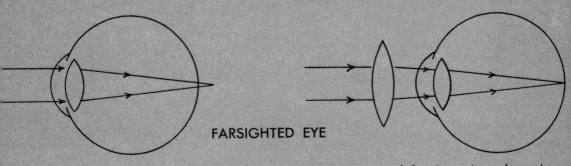

FARSIGHTED EYE

Image focused beyond Retina)

Corrected by Lens (eyeglasses)

Farsighted Eye (Presbyopia). This diagram of the farsighted eye shows the image focusing beyond the retina. This too can be readily corrected by appropriate eyeglasses.

Will wearing the proper eyeglasses lead to an improvement in farsightedness?

It will not bring about a cure but will improve the vision.

Is it ever bad to wear eyeglasses for farsightedness?

No.

How early can children be fitted with eyeglasses for farsightedness?

Usually at three years of age.

How can the doctor detect farsightedness in small children?

By a special examination known as retinoscopy.

Why does farsightedness get worse as one gets older?

As one gets older, the muscles in the eye get weaker and the patient is less able to compensate for his defect by muscle contraction.

Should farsighted people spare their eyes from excessive reading?

This is not necessary if the patient wears proper eyeglasses.

Does watching television have any harmful effect on the eyes of farsighted people?

No.

When are contact lenses recommended for farsightedness?

Contact lenses are rarely recommended for farsightedness.

Is there any medication which can be given to help farsightedness?

No.

Is there any surgical procedure which can help farsightedness?

No.

Does farsightedness ever cause blindness?

No.

ASTIGMATISM

What is astigmatism?

A defect in the curvature of the cornea whereby there is an inequality preventing the light rays from hitting the retina at a point of common focus.

What produces astigmatism?

The manner in which the eyeballs grow.

How does a person know if he has astigmatism?

Astigmatic people are more prone to eyestrain and soon become aware that something is wrong.

What is the treatment for astigmatism?

The wearing of proper corrective glasses will relieve the symptoms and improve vision greatly.

Does astigmatism ever get better by itself?

No.

Can astigmatism lead to blindness?

No.

CONJUNCTIVITIS

What is conjunctivitis?

An inflammation of the conjunctiva, the thin membrane which covers the white part of the eyeball and the inner surface of the eyelids.

What can cause conjunctivitis?

An injury, an infection, or an allergy. Injury can be caused by exposure to sunlight, dust, or wind. Infection may be caused by a streptococcus, staphylococcus, gonococcus, or any other bacteria.

What are the symptoms of conjunctivitis?

The symptoms of the traumatic (injury) type are redness, itching, burning, and tearing of the eyes. The symptoms of the infectious type are the same as for traumatic conjunctivitis, plus the fact that there is a pus discharge from the eye. The symptoms of the allergic type are redness, burning, tearing, and itching of the eyes and lids, often accompanied by symptoms in the nose and throat.

What is the treatment for conjunctivitis?

For the traumatic type, mild astringent eye drops. For the infectious type, antibiotic eye drops. For the allergic type, antihistamine or cortisone eye drops.

Is conjunctivitis contagious?

Only the infectious type is contagious.

How can one prevent the spread of the contagious type of conjunctivitis?

By isolating the patient and having him use his own soap and towel.

How long does it take for conjunctivitis to get well?

Usually two to four days, if there are no complications.

Does permanent damage to eyesight result from conjunctivitis?

No, unless there are complications.

What is the most common complication of conjunctivitis?

An ulceration of the cornea, which may leave a scar obscuring vision to a greater or lesser degree.

If conjunctivitis is due to a gonorrheal infection, can it be cured?

Yes, by proper use of the antibiotic medications.

What is the treatment for gonorrheal conjunctivitis?

The use of penicillin eye drops.

What are the preventive measures to avoid gonorrheal conjunctivitis?

If one has gonorrhea, strict personal hygiene is essential! The hands must be kept away from the eyes and penicillin eye drops should be used prophylactically.

What is "pink eye"?

"Pink eye" is a very contagious type of infectious conjunctivitis caused by special bacteria.

What are the symptoms of "pink eye"?

The same as for any infectious conjunctivitis.

How is "pink eye" treated?

By eye drops, which will bring about a cure in two to three days.

Can "pink eye" permanently injure the eyes?

No.

LACERATIONS, ABRASIONS, ULCERATIONS, AND FOREIGN BODIES OF THE CORNEA

What is the first-aid treatment for a scratch or foreign body in the eye?

The use of anesthetic eye drops and a bandage to cover the eye. After anesthetizing the eye, a foreign body can usually be wiped away with sterile, moist cotton on a stick.

What should one do if this occurs late at night when the eye doctor is not available?

The use of the anesthetic drops and a patch will relieve the patient of pain and keep the eye clean until the patient can consult an eye doctor in the morning.

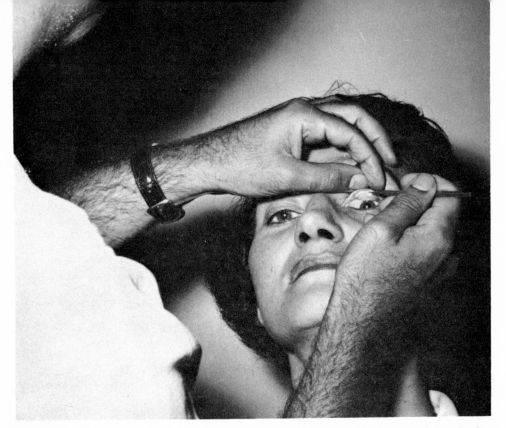

Removal of a Foreign Body—in this case a Cinder—from the Eye. Foreign bodies which cannot be easily and quickly removed should be treated by a physician. The cornea (the membrane over the pupil) may be scratched and infection may take place if untrained people attempt to remove firmly embedded foreign bodies.

Can serious damage to the eye result if one waits several hours before receiving medical treatment?

No, but one should not wait more than twelve hours before seeing a doctor.

What is the treatment for an abrasion (scratch) or ulcer of the cornea?

The use of antibiotic eye drops or ointment and a bandage to keep the eye covered. See your eye doctor.

Can a laceration of the cornea be successfully sutured?

Yes. This is done when there has been a deep or extensive laceration.

Is there any serious danger to the eye from a foreign body such as a small cinder or piece of steel?

If the foreign body is on the surface of the eye, there is usually very

403

little danger. If the foreign body has penetrated the eyeball, there is serious danger to the eye.

Do abrasions and lacerations tend to heal by themselves?

Small abrasions will heal by themselves. Lacerations usually have to be treated.

How does one prevent scar tissue from forming when abrasions or lacerations heal?

By the use of cortisone eye drops and the use of warm compresses to the eye.

Is impairment of vision often found after an injury of this type?

If a corneal abrasion is superficial and does not become infected, there is usually no impairment of vision. Intraocular foreign bodies very often result in impairment of vision.

How long do corneal abrasions take to heal?

With proper treatment, two to four days.

How long do corneal lacerations take to heal?

Usually two to three weeks.

What causes chronic ulceration of the cornea?

Chronic ulceration of the cornea occurs when the patient's resistance is low, as in diabetes or other debilitating illnesses.

What is the treatment for chronic or recurrent ulcers of the cornea?

The use of antibiotics, cauterization of the ulcer, and a bandage to keep the eye covered and safe from possible external contamination.

STYES AND CYSTS OF THE EYELIDS

What causes recurrent styes of the eyelids?

a. Lowered body resistance due to poor health.

b. Conjunctivitis (inflammation of the covering of the eye).

c. Blepharitis (inflammation of the eyelids).

d. Lack of cleanliness.

What is the treatment for styes?

Warm compresses and mild antiseptics will usually cause most of them to heal. Occasionally it is necessary for the eye surgeon to open them. Severe cases are treated with antibiotic drugs.

How long does it take for the usual stye to disappear?

About five to eight days.

What causes cysts of the eyelids (chalazion)?

An inflammation of one of the small glands in the lid, with a clogging of its opening to the surface.

What are the symptoms of a stye or cyst of the eyelid?

A markedly painful swelling and redness of the lid.

What is the treatment for chalazion?

Most of them will respond to warm compresses and eye drops. If they do not subside by themselves they must be opened and removed under local anesthesia in the ophthalmologist's office.

Do these cysts have a tendency to recur once they are cured?

No, but there is a tendency for people who have developed one cyst (chalazion) to develop others.

DACRYOCYSTITIS

What is dacryocystitis?

Dacryocystitis is an inflammation of the tear sac of the eye.

What causes dacryocystitis?

Dacryocystitis is usually secondary to a blocked tear canal.

405

What are the symptoms of dacryocystitis?

Severe pain and swelling of the inner corner of the eye, sometimes extending down toward the nose.

What is the treatment for dacryocystitis?

The use of antibiotics, and incision for drainage of pus.

Is recurrence frequent after cure of this condition?

Yes, unless the blockage of the tear canal is released by probing or by surgery.

How long does it take for someone with dacryocystitis to get well?

Usually, about a week.

IRITIS

What is iritis?

An inflammation of the iris, the colored part of the eyeball.

What causes iritis?

Iritis may be caused by local infection, tuberculosis, or syphilis.

What are the symptoms of iritis?

Pain, redness, and tearing of the eye, with inability to tolerate light.

What is the treatment for iritis?

The treatment will depend upon the cause of the disease. It will consist, usually, of eye drops containing atropine and cortisone.

Is recovery possible after iritis?

Yes, if treated early in its course.

Is the eyesight frequently damaged after iritis?

A severe iritis may leave permanent damage to vision.

How long does it take for iritis to get well?

One to two weeks.

GLAUCOMA

What is glaucoma?

A condition in which the pressure within the eyeball is elevated above normal.

What causes glaucoma?

The cause is unknown.

How often does glaucoma occur?

Two per cent of all adults over the age of forty will develop glaucoma.

Is it more common in males than in females?

No.

Does it occur in children?

There is a rare form of glaucoma in children which is present from birth. This is called congenital glaucoma.

Does glaucoma tend to run in families or to be inherited?

No.

What are the harmful effects of glaucoma?

If untreated, it will cause serious decrease in vision and may result in blindness.

What are the symptoms of glaucoma?

In the acute type, there is severe pain in the eye, redness of the eye, and blurring of vision. In the chronic type, the patient may have no symptoms whatever.

How can one tell if he has glaucoma?

In the acute type, he will know very quickly because of the severe pain and blurring of vision. In the chronic type, it may be discovered on routine eye examination by the ophthalmologist.

Is there any way to prevent getting glaucoma?

If the eye doctor suspects the patient of being a potential glaucoma case, he may prescribe prophylactic eye drops which will protect against the disease.

What tests are performed to make the diagnosis of glaucoma?

a. Taking the pressure of the eyeball with an instrument known as a tonomoter.
b. Checking the visual fields.
c. Performing provocative tests.

Does glaucoma usually affect both eyes at the same time?

No, but a patient who has developed the condition in one eye is more prone to develop it in the other eye at some later date.

What is the treatment for glaucoma?

In the acute type, eye drops are used to reduce the intraocular pressure. If the pressure cannot be reduced after eight hours, surgery is indicated. In the chronic type, eye drops may be continued for years as the sole means of treatment, provided the pressure remains controlled; otherwise surgery is necessary.

Is hospitalization necessary, or can the patient be satisfactorily treated at home?

Hospital care is necessary if surgery has to be done.

Is surgery always necessary?

It depends upon the pressure and the visual fields. If these can be controlled by eye drops, surgery will not be necessary.

What will happen if surgery is not performed when indicated?

Blindness will result.

What will happen if the eye drops are not used when indicated?

The patient may eventually lose the sight of the involved eye.

Does glaucoma clear up by itself without treatment?

Usually not.

Is the surgery for glaucoma dangerous?

No.

What are the chances for recovery after surgery?

In the acute type, the chances are excellent. In the chronic type, the earlier surgery is done, the better the chances for a good result.

What kind of operation is performed?

An iridectomy, wherein a small piece of the iris is removed to allow drainage and to lessen the pressure within the eyeball. The actual procedure varies from case to case, depending upon whether the surgeon is dealing with an acute or a chronic glaucoma.

What anesthetic is used?

Local anesthesia.

How long a hospital stay is necessary?

Usually, five to seven days.

Are special private nurses required after surgery?

No.

Is there a visible scar after glaucoma operations?

No, except that one can see where a small piece of iris has been removed.

Does glaucoma recur after it has been operated upon?

Usually not in the acute type. In the chronic glaucoma, it may recur.

What limitations on activity are imposed after a successful glaucoma operation?

None.

409

How soon after the operation can one do the following:

Bathe	One week.
Walk out in the street	One week.
Walk up and down stairs	One week.
Perform household duties	Three to four weeks.
Drive a car	Four weeks.
Resume marital relations	Six weeks.
Return to work	Four weeks.
Resume all physical activities	Four weeks.

Is it necessary to return for periodic examinations after an attack o glaucoma?

Yes. The physician will pay particular attention to the health of th uninvolved eye.

CATARACT

What is a cataract?

An opacity or a clouding of the lens.

Where is the lens of the eye?

It is located inside the eye, just behind the pupil.

What is its function?

To focus the image on to the retina in the back of the eye.

What happens when a patient has a cataract?

The opaque lens does not allow light to enter the eyeball. Vision i thereby decreased.

What causes cataract?

The cause is usually unknown. Sometimes, however, it may be du to diabetes, a glandular disorder, an infection within the eyeball or a direct injury to the lens.

Do cataracts tend to run in families or to be inherited?

Occasionally one finds that a tendency toward cataract formation is inherited.

What harm results from leaving a cataract untreated?

As cataracts progress, vision decreases. If a cataract of long standing is not removed, it will become overripe, causing a severe inflammation and possible loss of the eyeball.

How can one tell if he has a cataract?

Cataracts should be suspected if there is blurring of vision which cannot be improved by glasses. In the later stages it is possible to see the cataract as a white opacity in the pupil.

Do cataracts usually affect both eyes at the same time?

No, but a person who has had a cataract is more prone to develop one on the other eye at some later date.

Is there any way to prevent getting cataract?

No.

What tests are performed to make a positive diagnosis of cataract?

By using an instrument called an ophthalmoscope, the opacity of the lens can be seen readily.

What is the treatment for cataract?

Surgical removal of the lens.

At what stage should a cataract be removed?

When it is ripe. This usually does not take place until the vision in the involved eye is markedly diminished. However, an unripe cataract may be removed in certain cases, if the patient's vision is too poor to allow him to do his work.

Do cataracts ever disappear by themselves?

No.

What are the chances for recovery following cataract surgery?

In over 90 per cent of cases, good results are obtained.

How long does an operation for removal of cataracts take to perform?

Forty to sixty minutes.

What kind of operation is performed?

An incision is made at the margin of the cornea and the white of the eye. Through this incision, the surgeon inserts an instrument, grasp the lens, and removes it.

What anesthetic is used?

Usually a local anesthetic.

How long a hospital stay is necessary for a cataract operation?

Four to six days.

Are special preoperative examinations necessary before a cataract operation?

It is important to know that the patient is in good general health and free from infection, diabetes, etc. Poor general health or a distant focus of infection will interfere with the result of a cataract operation.

Are special private nurses required after surgery?

It is advisable to have private nurses for the first forty-eight hours.

Is the postoperative period especially painful?

No.

What is the postoperative treatment following cataract surgery?

The patient is kept flat on his back for the first forty-eight hours with *both* eyes bandaged. After this, the unoperated eye is exposed and the patient is allowed to move around in bed.

What are possible complications of cataract surgery?

Infection or hemorrhage within the eyeball.

How are these complications treated?

Infections are treated by the use of antibiotics. Hemorrhage is treated by applying a pressure bandage to the eyeball and keeping the patient quiet in bed.

How long does it take for the wound to heal after the usual cataract operation?

One to two weeks.

What kind of scar remains?

The scar is practically invisible.

Do cataracts ever recur once they have been removed?

Occasionally, a membrane may form and obscure vision. However, this can be removed by a rather simple operation, and good vision will result.

How soon may a patient obtain glasses after a cataract operation?

Within one month. If vision in the unoperated eye is good, it is sometimes not possible to use glasses for the operated eye, as the patient may see double.

What postoperative precautions must be followed?

The patient should not bend over or do strenuous work for about one month after a cataract removal.

After recovery from a cataract operation, does one return to a completely normal existence?

Yes.

How soon after a cataract operation can one do the following:

Bathe	Two weeks.
Walk in the street	One week.
Walk up and down stairs	Two weeks.
Perform household duties	Four weeks.
Drive a car	Six weeks.

Resume marital relations   Twelve weeks.

Return to light work   Four weeks.

Return to heavy work   Eight weeks.

Resume all physical activities   Twelve weeks.

STRABISMUS
(Crossed Eyes)

What is strabismus?

A condition in which the eyes are not straight but are crossed. One or both eyes may turn in or out. The condition may be inconstant or constant.

What causes strabismus?

When strabismus is noticed at birth, it is due either to small brain hemorrhages or to abnormal attachments of the muscles of the eyeball. When it occurs after the first or second year of life, it is usually due to a weakness of the "fusion center" in the brain. It may also be associated with a weak or paralyzed eye muscle.

Convergent strabismus, where the eye turns in, is usually associated with farsightedness. Divergent strabismus, where the eye turns out, is usually associated with nearsightedness.

Does strabismus tend to run in families or to be inherited?

Yes, occasionally.

What is meant by "a cast in the eye"?

This is another term for crossed eyes.

Is it more difficult to cure eyes that turn out than eyes that turn in?

Yes.

How early in life can crossed eyes be recognized?

Often, at birth. Definitely, at some time during the first three years of life.

What percentage of crossed eyes can be cured with medical treatment alone?

Fifty to 60 per cent.

What is the medical treatment?

The wearing of proper glasses and the performance of prescribed eye exercises. Often, the wearing of a patch over the good eye will prove helpful.

How long must one wear glasses before the eyes straighten?

If the eyes are going to straighten, it will occur after the glasses are worn for six months.

Why does strabismus sometimes not improve even after glasses are worn?

Because it is due to some factor other than nearsightedness or farsightedness, such as faulty attachments of the muscles surrounding the eyeballs.

What is the earliest age at which a child will be able to wear glasses for crossed eyes?

Two years of age.

What harm results from strabismus?

It is disfiguring and can produce deep psychological harm. Convergent strabismus, if not treated, may result in poor vision or even loss of vision in the eye that turns in.

Is there any way to prevent strabismus?

Yes. If the patient shows signs of developing strabismus, the wearing of proper eyeglasses will often straighten the eye.

What is the treatment for strabismus?

The wearing of proper eyeglasses. Occasionally, eye drops are beneficial. If, after a patient has worn eyeglasses for six months, a bad strabismus has not improved, surgery is indicated.

Is there any way to prevent eyes that turn in from developing poor vision?

Yes. The patient wears a patch over the good eye, which forces him to use the weak eye. This will very often improve the vision in the weak eye.

Is surgery always necessary for strabismus?

No. If the strabismus is mild and inconstant, surgery is not necessary.

Does strabismus ever get well by itself without treatment?

Yes. A mild case may get well by itself.

What are the risks of surgery for strabismus?

The risks are practically nil.

What are the chances for a good result from surgery?

The chances for a good cosmetic result are excellent.

How long does it take to perform an operation for strabismus?

This will depend upon the number of muscles that have to be operated upon. The average case takes one hour.

Eye Muscles. This diagram shows the muscle attachments to the outside of the eyeball. When these muscles fail to function normally, the eyes may become crossed or they may diverge. Both conditions can be helped greatly by surgery. The surgeon will either shorten or lengthen the muscles in order to bring the eyes into proper alignment. Such an operation, although delicate, is not very complicated and may be performed safely on small children.

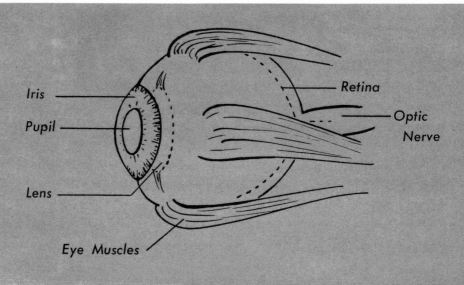

Iris — Pupil — Lens — Eye Muscles — Retina — Optic Nerve

What kind of operation is performed?

This will vary with the type of strabismus. It may be necessary to strengthen a muscle. This is done by cutting off a piece of the muscle, or shortening it, and reattaching it to its original insertion on the eyeball. It may be necessary to weaken a muscle. This is done by detaching it from its insertion and reattaching it further back on the eyeball.

What anesthetic is used?

For children, a general anesthetic. For adults, a local anesthetic.

How long a hospital stay is necessary?

One to two days.

Are special preoperative treatments necessary?

No.

Are special private nurses required after surgery?

No.

Is the postoperative period exceptionally painful?

No.

What special postoperative procedures are carried out?

Occasionally, eye drops are necessary following surgery. If the eyes are not absolutely straight, it may be necessary for the patient to take special eye exercises. These exercises are known as orthoptics.

How long does it take for the wound to heal following a strabismus operation?

About two weeks.

Do patients ever see double after a strabismus operation?

Yes, but this condition usually disappears within three to four weeks.

What kind of scar remains after this operation?

The scar is invisible.

417

Does strabismus ever recur after it has been operated upon?

Only once in a great while.

What postoperative precautions must be followed?

For about one week after surgery, the patient should not read or watch television.

Is it necessary for a patient to continue wearing glasses after surgery?

If the patient was nearsighted or farsighted before the operation, it will be necessary for him to continue wearing glasses. Strabismus operations do not cure these eye conditions.

After full recovery from a strabismus operation, can one use his eyes as much as he wishes?

Yes.

How soon after a strabismus operation can one do the following?

Bathe	Two weeks.
Walk in the street	One week.
Walk up and down stairs	One week.
Resume some physical activity	Seven to ten days.
Perform light household duties	Three to four weeks.
Perform heavy household duties	Four to five weeks.

DETACHED RETINA

Where is the retina located and what is its function?

The retina lines the inside of the back two-thirds of the eyeball. It is the sensitive part of the eyeball which transforms the light impulses into nerve impulses and transmits them to the brain.

What is detachment of the retina?

A condition in which the retina is pulled away from its attachments to the inside of the eyeball.

What causes detached retina?

It may be caused by an injury, inflammation, extreme nearsighted-ness, or a tumor of the choroid (a portion of the eye lying beneath the retina).

Does detached retina occur more often among men than women?

No.

Does it tend to run in families or to be inherited?

No.

What harm results from a detached retina?

A detached retina, if not treated, may result in blindness.

How can one tell if he has a detached retina?

A detached retina may be suspected if there is a veil before the eyes or blurred vision in one portion of the eyeball.

Is there any way to prevent getting a detached retina?

Exceptionally nearsighted people should be particularly careful to guard against injuries to the head.

What tests are performed to make a positive diagnosis of detached retina?

The eye specialist will examine the eye with an ophthalmoscope, which allows him to see the retina. In the early cases, where the detachment is slight, or where the detachment is not centrally located, several examinations may be required before a definite diagnosis can be made.

What is the treatment for detached retina?

Two types of operations can be performed. In one type, an electric needle is applied to the outer surface of the eyeball over the area of the detached retina. This sets up an inflammation and inflam-matory reaction within the eyeball. As the inflammation subsides, adhesions form, which pull the retina back into its normal position. The second type of operation involves the removal of a section of the wall of the eyeball, thus decreasing the size of the eyeball and allowing the retina to assume its normal position.

What will happen if surgery is not performed?

The eye will become blind.

What are the chances for recovery?

In over 50 per cent of the cases, recovery takes place. This will depend upon how long the detachment has been present and upon its extent and severity.

How long does it take to perform an operation for detached retina?

Approximately one hour.

What anesthetic is used in surgery for retinal detachment?

Local anesthesia. However, general anesthesia may be used in certain cases.

How long a hospital stay is necessary?

Three to six weeks. It takes a while for the retina to reattach itself and become firmly adherent to its underlying structures.

Is the postoperative period exceptionally painful?

No.

What special postoperative treatments are carried out?

For four days the patient is usually kept flat on his back with both eyes bandaged. After this, the unoperated eye is exposed. The operated eye is kept bandaged from four to six weeks, and after this period the patient uses pinhole spectacles in order to limit the motion of the eyeball.

How long does it take for the wound to heal?

Three to six weeks.

Are postoperative precautions necessary?

Yes. The patient must limit physical activity for about two months.

Does detachment ever recur after it has once been successfully treated?

Occasionally.

After full recovery from a detached retina, can one return to a completely normal existence?

Yes.

How soon after surgery for detached retina can one do the following:

Bathe	Three weeks.
Walk out in the street	Two weeks.
Walk up and down stairs	Four to six weeks.
Perform light household duties	Eight weeks.
Perform heavy household duties	Eight to twelve weeks.
Drive a car	Six weeks.
Resume all physical activities	Twelve weeks.

When should one return for a checkup after an operation for detached retina?

Monthly for the first three months; thereafter, every four to six months.

TUMORS OF THE EYE

How common are tumors within the eyeball?

They are rare.

What are the common types of tumors within the eyeball?

a. Sarcomas, which arise in the choroid.
b. Gliomas, which arise in the retina.

What age groups are most prone to develop these tumors?

The glioma of the retina usually occurs in children under the age of five. It occurs in one eye in most cases, but sometimes occurs in both eyes. The sarcoma of the choroid usually occurs in adults between the ages of forty and sixty and involves one eye only.

421

What causes tumors of the eye?

The cause is unknown.

What are the symptoms of glioma in children?

If the child is very young, he may not complain at all. The parent, however, may notice a peculiar yellow color in the pupil. Older children may complain of blurring of vision. In adults, there may be blurring of vision. However, some patients may have no symptoms, and the condition is recognized only on routine examination by the eye specialist.

What is the treatment for glioma when only one eye is involved?

The eyeball should be removed as soon as possible! If both eyes are involved, the eye with the larger tumor is usually removed and the tumor in the other eye is treated with x-ray and radium.

What will happen if the operation is not performed?

The condition will spread to other parts of the body and cause death.

What are the chances of recovery in adults?

The chances for recovery are good.

What are the chances for recovery when children have eye tumors?

Eye tumors in children are very serious. However, latest reports are encouraging, and more and more children are being saved.

RETINAL THROMBOSIS

What is retinal thrombosis?

A condition in which clots form within the retinal blood vessels. As a result, a hemorrhage of the retina takes place, and vision is blurred or lost.

What causes retinal thrombosis?

It is associated with hardening or arteriosclerosis of the blood vessels.

What are the symptoms of retinal thrombosis?

Abrupt blurring or loss of vision.

What is the treatment for retinal thrombosis?

In mild cases, rest of the eyes is all that is required. In severe cases, medication to reduce the clotting of the blood may be necessary.

Does recovery take place after retinal thrombosis?

In mild cases, yes. Severe cases may result in blindness.

How long is one sick with retinal thrombosis?

In mild cases, four to six weeks. Chronic cases may keep recurring until there is loss of vision.

SYMPATHETIC OPHTHALMIA

What is sympathetic ophthalmia?

A strange inflammation which affects the healthy eye after an injury to the other eye.

What causes sympathetic ophthalmia?

The cause is unknown.

How does one know if sympathetic ophthalmia is developing?

If a patient has an injured eye which is red and painful, and he then develops redness or blurring of vision in the opposite eye, he should consult the eye specialist immediately.

Is there any way to prevent sympathetic ophthalmia from developing?

In the past, it was often necessary to remove the injured eye in order to save the vision in the opposite eye. Today, the use of cortisone and the antibiotic drugs often prevents sympathetic ophthalmia from developing in the uninjured eye.

After sympathetic ophthalmia has set in, is there any chance for complete recovery?

Yes, but not very often.

TRACHOMA

What is trachoma?

A serious specific chronic inflammation of the eyes. It involves the cornea, the conjunctiva, and the eyelids.

What causes trachoma?

The cause of trachoma is unknown, but poor hygiene and diet seem to play a great part in its causation.

Where is trachoma most likely to be encountered?

In Eastern Europe and Northern Africa.

What are the symptoms of trachoma?

In early cases, the symptoms are redness and tearing of the eyes. If the cornea is involved, there will be pain and extreme sensitivity to light.

What is the treatment for trachoma?

The use of the sulfa drugs has proved to be effective in the early stages of the disease.

Does trachoma ever cause blindness?

In serious cases, yes.

Can trachoma be cured?

Yes, in its early stages.

How long does trachoma last?

The neglected cases may last a lifetime.

How can trachoma be prevented?

    a. By proper diet and good hygiene.
    b. By avoiding contact with people with trachoma.
    c. By prompt medical attention to any eye irritation in those who live in an area where trachoma is prevalent.

23 *The Female Organs*

MENSTRUATION

What is menstruation?

It is a bloody discharge from the vagina occurring at more or less regular intervals throughout the childbearing period of a woman's life. Each month the womb (uterus) prepares itself for pregnancy by certain changes in its lining membrane. If a fertilized egg does not implant itself into the wall of the uterus, its lining disintegrates and is discharged from the uterus in the form of the menstrual flow.

When does menstruation begin?

Some time between the ages of eleven and sixteen years. This will depend upon factors such as climate, race, and general health. In rare instances, normal menstruation may commence before the eleventh year and after the sixteenth year.

How long does menstruation last?

It usually continues until age forty-five to fifty-five.

What is the normal interval between menstrual periods?

The normal menstrual cycle occurs approximately every twenty-eight days. However, this is very variable and some women may develop a cycle with intervals of twenty-one, thirty, thirty-five, or even forty days. The important thing to note is a *change* in the menstrual

425

cycle. A girl who menstruates every twenty-eight days and then changes to a twenty-one-day cycle or a thirty-five-day cycle should consult her physician.

What are common conditions, other than pregnancy, which will cause a woman to miss a period?
   a. A sudden change in climate.
   b. An acute emotional upset.
   c. An acute infection or illness.
   d. Hormone imbalance or poor function of the endocrine glands.
   e. A cyst or tumor of the ovary.
   f. Poor nutrition or vitamin deficiency.
   g. Marked anemia.
   h. Chronic debilitating diseases, such as tuberculosis, cancer, etc.
   i. The onset of menopause (change of life).

How soon after a period has been missed can it be determined if pregnancy exists?

A pregnancy test can give this information approximately fourteen days after a period has been missed. (See Chapter 53, on Pregnancy and Childbirth.)

Can medications, or other artificial measures, be used successfully to bring on a menstrual period when it has been skipped because of pregnancy?

No. Hot baths, laxatives, or patent drugs will not bring on a period if pregnancy exists.

Are there harmful effects from taking medications to bring on a menstrual period when it is late?

Yes. The patient should never treat herself to bring on a menstrual period artificially. There is definite danger from the use of such medications.

How long do menstrual periods usually last?

Approximately four to five days. Here again, the length of time may vary from one to seven or eight days. The important consideration is a deviation from the usual duration.

What is the natural appearance of menstrual blood?

Normal menstrual blood is a pink to dark-red color and does not clot. The presence of clots, or pieces of blood, or marked change in the amount of flow or the duration of the period should warrant medical consultation.

Is there a detectable odor to normal menstruation?

No.

Is it normal for some women to have slight swelling of the face, neck, breasts, and abdomen during the menstrual period?

Yes.

What is the significance of scant menstruation?

a. If pregnancy is not a likelihood, then a single instance of scant menstruation should be disregarded as insignificant.

b. Repeated, persistent scant menstruation is often due to a failure of the bleeding mechanism caused either by an upset in the glands which regulate menstruation (such as the pituitary or the ovaries or the thyroid), or by an abnormal condition within the uterus itself.

c. In women in their forties or early fifties, scant menstruation may be the forerunner of change of life (menopause).

What is the cause of failure of onset of menstruation?

This is almost always caused by a disturbance in glandular function.

Should lack of menstruation in a girl in her middle or late teens warrant investigation by a physician?

Yes. Proper treatment frequently can correct this condition.

What is the treatment for scant menstruation?

During the childbearing age, scant menstruation requires no treatment if there is evidence that the woman is ovulating regularly. This means that she is producing a mature egg from an ovary each month.

If ovulation is not taking place, further medical investigation is indicated. This should include an evaluation of the activity of the various endocrine glands. Where a deficiency in the secretion of a particular hormone is discovered, specific treatment is directed toward replacing or correcting such deficiency.

Does the giving of the appropriate hormone usually correct scant menstruation or absent menstruation?

When properly administered, hormone treatments will usually bring about regulation of the normal cycle.

Does scant menstruation prevent pregnancy from taking place?

Only when it is associated with lack of ovulation. If ovulation is present, scant menstruation will not interfere with pregnancy.

Does scant menstruation often indicate the beginning of menopause in a woman in her late thirties, forties, or fifties?

Yes.

What is the significance of irregular menstrual bleeding?

Its significance varies with the type of irregularity. Most women have a slight variation of one to two days, either in onset or in length of flow. Marked changes in the time of onset, in the length of the flow, the amount of bleeding, or the presence of bleeding not associated with menstruation requires investigation by the gynecologist. The appearance of "staining" just before or just after menstruation should also be investigated.

What are some of the more common causes of irregular menstruation?

a. Infection within the female genital system.

b. A benign tumor of the uterus or ovaries.

c. A malignant tumor of the uterus or ovaries.

d. Imbalance of the endocrine glands (pituitary, thyroid, or ovaries).

e. Ectopic pregnancy (a pregnancy which takes place outside of the uterus, usually in the Fallopian tubes).

What is the significance of excessive menstrual bleeding?

Excessive bleeding during the period is not normal and should be investigated. It may be indicative of infection, glandular upset, or the presence of a tumor within the uterus or the ovaries.

What is the treatment for excessive menstrual bleeding?

This will depend entirely upon the cause; each will be discussed separately in other sections of this chapter.

What is dysmenorrhea?

This term applies to painful menstruation. There are two essential types:

a. Primary dysmenorrhea, in which there are no demonstrable evidences of disease.

b. Secondary dysmenorrhea, in which the pain is associated with an organic disease within the pelvis.

What causes primary dysmenorrhea?

The exact cause is unknown. However, one of the more important factors associated with this condition is the emotional make-up of the individual. Low pain thresholds, poor psychological orientation toward menstruation, a painful emotional experience related to menstruation, or an abnormal reaction toward the idea of pregnancy is often noted in women who have this condition.

What is the treatment for primary dysmenorrhea?

The first approach should be directed toward greater understanding of the emotional problems facing the patient. In addition to these measures, medications such as the antispasmodic drugs, vitamins, diuretic drugs, or the administration of female or male hormones may bring about relief.

Is surgery ever helpful in treating painful menstruation?

If the dysmenorrhea is so severe that it becomes disabling, surgery may be contemplated. This will consist of an abdominal operation (presacral neurectomy) in which a nerve supplying the uterus is severed.

Is presacral neurectomy often advocated?

No. It is undertaken only as a last resort if other measures fail to relieve painful menstruation.

What are the common causes of secondary dysmenorrhea?

a. Inflammation of the tubes or ovaries.
b. Fibroids or polyps of the uterus or cervix.
c. Endometriosis. (See the section on the Uterus in this chapter.)
d. Congestion or varicose veins within the pelvic structures.

What is the treatment for secondary dysmenorrhea?

Since the causes are associated with pelvic disease, secondary dysmenorrhea can be cured only by removing the underlying disease process. Until such time as this is carried out, relief may be obtained by the giving of pain-relieving and antispasmodic drugs, hormones, and diuretics.

Is dysmenorrhea cured by pregnancy?

Usually not. Pregnancy will alleviate dysmenorrhea only for the duration of the pregnancy.

Is it wise for women to go to bed or otherwise treat themselves as invalids when they have a painful menstrual period?

This should be avoided whenever possible. The best attitude toward menstruation should be to continue normal activity insofar as it is possible. Pampering will only tend to make the symptoms worse.

What is premenstrual tension?

It is the periodic appearance of disturbing anxieties occurring about the middle of the menstrual cycle and increasing in intensity as menstruation approaches. This tension subsides when menstruation begins.

What causes premenstrual tension?

The exact cause is unknown, but this phenomenon is attributed to a change in the amount of hormones which are secreted at various times throughout the menstrual cycle.

What are some of the symptoms of premenstrual tension?

In severe cases, there may be personality changes, irritability, emotional instability, episodes of crying, etc. Physical symptoms, such as backache, severe abdominal cramps, breast pain and tenderness, headaches, swelling of the legs, are some of the more definable features.

What is the treatment for premenstrual tension?

Simple measures will include:

a. Restriction of salt intake prior to menstruation.

b. The giving of medications to increase the output of urine and the reduction of tissue fluids.

c. The taking of female hormones.

d. The use of male hormones in small doses.

Will the giving of male sex hormones to women with menstrual disorders cause excessive hair to grow or the voice to change or masculine characteristics to develop?

No! The amount of male hormone given for these disorders is not nearly sufficient to produce such changes. Where large doses are needed, male characteristics may appear but will disappear immediately upon discontinuing medication.

Are tampons which are inserted into the vagina harmful to use?

No.

What is the normal number of sanitary napkins required each day during a menstrual period?

This varies markedly for each individual. The only important consideration is a variation from the usual number used.

Should a young child of ten or eleven years be told about menstruation?

Yes. Truthfully preparing the girl for menstruation is a very important parental duty. Children should not be permitted to reach the age of menstruation without adequate advance information.

431

Is it true that if a mother has painful menstruation her child will develop it?

Painful menstruation is not inherited, but a child unconsciously tends to mimic her mother's reactions. It is wise, therefore, for the mother to minimize the discomfort of menstruation.

Can a shower be taken with safety during a menstrual period?

Yes.

Is it dangerous to go swimming or to take a bath during a menstrual period?

No.

Are marital relations dangerous or harmful during menstruation?

No, but many married people avoid this practice.

THE EXTERNAL GENITALS

What is the vulva?

It is the area that surrounds the entrance to the vagina, and is composed of the clitoris, the labia majora (major lips), the labia minora (the minor lips), the opening of the urethra from the bladder, the hymen, the Bartholin glands, and the opening of the vagina.

What is the clitoris and what is its function?

It is a small knoblike structure on top of the vaginal opening where the lips of the vulva join together. The clitoris is a focal point of sexual excitement and plays an important part in marital relations. The tissue structure of the clitoris is quite similar to that of the male penis.

What is the hymen?

It is a fold of mucous membrane which partially or completely covers the vaginal opening. It is this membrane which is ruptured on first sexual contact.

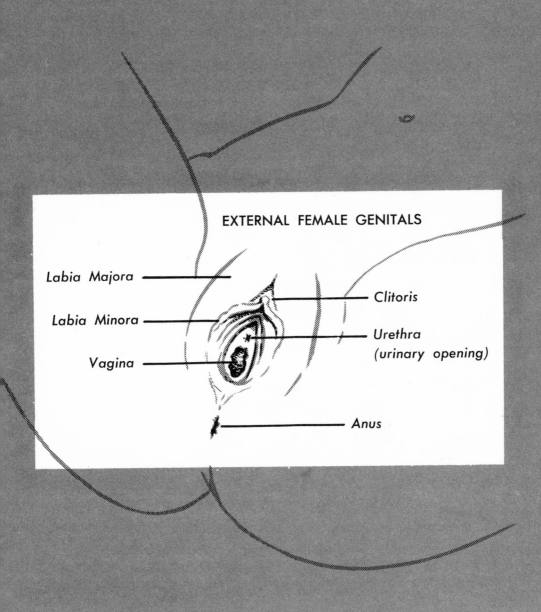

EXTERNAL FEMALE GENITALS

Labia Majora ————————

Labia Minora ————————

Vagina ————————

———————— Clitoris

———————— Urethra
(urinary opening)

———————— Anus

The External Female Genitals. This diagram shows the female external genitals, including the clitoris, the lips of the vagina, and the vagina. It is amazing how few females are familiar with their own bodily construction in this region.

Are there many variations in the structure of the hymen?

Yes. In most girls, the hymen is not a complete covering but contains perforations which permit the exit of the menstrual flow. Rarely, these perforations are missing and the hymen must be incised surgically in order to permit the exit of menstrual blood.

What is a hymenotomy?

The surgical incision of the hymen in order to enlarge the vaginal opening.

Why is hymenotomy performed?

a. For an imperforate hymen.

b. At the time of marriage, when a thickened or rigid hymenal ring makes sexual intercourse difficult or impossible.

Is hymenotomy a major operative procedure?

No. It is a simple procedure performed under light anesthesia in the hospital.

Is hymenotomy always necessary when intercourse is difficult?

No. Most cases of painful intercourse are due to vaginal spasm. This spasm is brought about by tension and fear of sexual relations. By proper advice and instruction, newly married women can overcome many of their fears, thus controlling the spasm.

Is difficulty in breaking the hymen a common occurrence?

No. It is relatively rare.

How soon after hymenotomy can marital relations be attempted?

About three to four weeks.

What is the cause of painful intercourse in women who have been having normal relations for many years?

a. An emotional problem is often responsible for painful intercourse (dyspareunia) when it appears later in married life.

b. Less commonly, there is an organic condition, such as an inflammation of the vagina or an inflammation of the pelvic organs, which is responsible for painful intercourse.

What are the Bartholin glands?

They are two small, bulblike structures located in the lower end of the lips, one on each side of the vagina. They are connected to the vaginal canal by a narrow duct.

What is the function of the Bartholin glands?

They secrete a mucous substance which acts as a lubricant for the inner surface of the lips of the vagina.

What is a Bartholin cyst?

It is a swelling of the duct, or the duct and the gland, caused by a blockage at the vaginal end of the duct. These cysts may be as small as a pea or as large as a plum.

What are the usual symptoms of a Bartholin cyst?

a. Pain on walking or during intercourse.

b. A swelling in the lips (labia).

What is the treatment for a Bartholin cyst?

Either surgical removal or incision into the cyst and fashioning a new opening (marsupialization operation).

Is hospitalization necessary for this type of operation?

Yes, for three to five days.

What is a Bartholin abscess?

It is an infection of a Bartholin gland caused either by gonorrhea or other bacteria.

What is the treatment for a Bartholin abscess?

a. Antibiotic drugs, hot soaks, and sedatives for the relief of pain.

b. In the more severe case, it will be necessary to incise and drain the abscess or to create a new permanent opening by performing a "marsupialization" operation.

Is hospitalization necessary for incision and drainage of a Bartholin abscess?

Yes. This procedure must be carried out under general anesthesia and will require hospitalization for a few days. In some instances, under local anesthesia, incision and drainage are performed as an office procedure.

Is there any other form of treatment for a Bartholin abscess?

Yes. Electric fulguration is often carried out after incision and drainage. This will destroy the lining membrane of the abscess and may bring about a cure.

What is vulvitis?

It is an inflammation or infection of the area about the external genitals. It is most often associated with an infection within the vagina.

What is leukoplakia of the vulva?

It is a disease of the skin of the vulva characterized by an overgrowth of cells and a tendency toward the formation of cancer. The areas of leukoplakia look grayish-white and develop a parchment-like appearance.

What causes leukoplakia of the vulva?

The exact cause is unknown, but it is supposedly related to a decrease in the secretion of ovarian hormone which takes place after menopause.

Who is most likely to develop leukoplakia?

Women who have passed the menopause.

Is leukoplakia of the vulva a common condition?

No. It is relatively infrequent.

What are the symptoms of leukoplakia of the vulva?

Itching is the most striking feature of this condition. Scratching will often lead to secondary infection from surface bacteria and may lead to inflammation, swelling, pain, redness, and even bleeding from the vicinity.

Does leukoplakia ever develop into cancer of the vulva?

Yes. It is estimated that about 25 per cent of the cases of cancer of the vulva originated from leukoplakia. However, this does not mean that all women with leukoplakia will develop cancer.

What is the treatment for leukoplakia of the vulva?

a. If infection is present, antibiotic drugs should be given locally and orally.
b. If itching is severe, anesthetic ointments should be applied.
c. Ovarian hormones should be given to forestall the progress of the disease.
d. Because of its pre-cancerous nature, surgical removal of the involved tissues is often carried out.

Does leukoplakia ever clear up by itself?

Temporary relief often results from medical management, but surgery is the only real cure for this condition.

How long does it usually take for leukoplakia to develop into cancer?

This is a very slow process which takes place over a period of years. There is, therefore, plenty of time to eradicate the lesions before they undergo malignant changes.

Does cancer ever involve the vulva?

Yes. The clitoris, the lips, the Bartholin glands, or the opening of the urethra may sometimes be involved in a cancerous process.

Is there any way to prevent cancer of the vulva?

Yes, by thorough surgical treatment of leukoplakia.

What is the treatment for cancer of the vulva?

Vulvectomy. This means the surgical removal of all those structures comprising the vulva. The lymph glands in the groin are also removed in performing a radical vulvectomy for the eradication of an extensive cancer of the vulva.

Is cancer of the vulva curable?

Yes, if treated properly in its early stages by vulvectomy. It is estimated that more than 60 per cent of cancers of the vulva can be cured permanently.

How is the diagnosis of cancer of the vulva made?

A piece of tissue is removed surgically and submitted to microscopic examination.

What is the incidence of cancer of the vulva?

It is estimated that cancer of the vulva constitutes about 2 to 3 per cent of all cancers affecting the female organs.

Who is most likely to develop cancer of the vulva?

Women beyond sixty years of age.

Is vulvectomy a serious operation?

Yes, but operative recovery takes place in almost all cases.

What is the vagina?

It is a tubelike canal, approximately three to four inches in length, extending internally from its opening at the vulva to the cervix of the uterus. It is lined by a mucous membrane which has many folds and great elasticity.

What are the functions of the vagina?

    a. It is the ultimate female organ of intercourse.
    b. It is a receptacle for the deposit of male sperm.
    c. It is the outlet for the discharge of menstrual fluid.
    d. It is the passageway for delivery of the baby during labor.

Should women douche regularly?

Douching should be reserved for conditions accompanied by vaginal discharge, odor, or other symptoms.

What is the best solution with which to douche?

An acid douche containing white distilled vinegar or lactic acid.

Are strong antiseptic douches harmful?

Yes. Strong chemicals can cause vaginal ulcers or burns.

Should young girls douche if they have a vaginal discharge or unpleasant odor?

Not without a gynecologist's specific instructions.

Should women take a cleansing douche the day following marital relations or following the conclusion of a menstrual period?

Yes, as it will often prevent unpleasant odor or discharge.

Is cancer of the vagina very common?

No. This is a very rare disease.

What is the treatment for cancer of the vagina?

a. Wide surgical excision of the vagina or radium implantation.

What other growths may affect the vagina?

a. Polyps.
b. Cysts.
c. Benign tumors, such as fibromas of the vaginal wall.

What is the treatment for benign growths of the vagina?

Simple surgical removal will bring about a cure in all of the above conditions.

What is prolapse of the uterus?

It is an abnormal descent of the uterus and cervix into the vagina. It is often associated with disturbance of the bladder and the rectum.

What causes prolapse of the uterus?

Most cases occur as a result of stretching or tears which have been incurred during labor and delivery. Women who have had several children may suffer stretching or tearing of the ligaments and muscles which ordinarily support the uterus and the vagina.

Is prolapse of the uterus caused by poor obstetrical management?

No. Tears of supporting ligaments may take place despite excellent obstetrical care.

439

Are there various degrees of prolapse?

Yes. There may be just slight descent of the uterus and cervix into the vagina, or the entire cervix and uterus may come down so far that they appear outside the vaginal opening.

What are the symptoms of prolapse of the uterus?

There is a feeling of fullness in the vagina and a sensation that something is falling down. These symptoms are aggravated after walking or lifting a heavy object. The prolapsed structures may interfere with sexual intercourse and a disturbance in urination and bowel function may be present. Symptoms will depend largely upon the degree of prolapse.

Can prolapse of the uterus be prevented?

Good obstetrical care will tend to minimize the incidence of prolapse, but it often cannot prevent it.

What is the treatment for prolapse?

The treatment is surgical. It will require a plastic operation upon the vagina to reconstruct the ligaments and muscles or, in a woman past the menopause, it may require the removal of the uterus and cervix (vaginal hysterectomy).

Are operations for prolapse serious?

They are considered major surgery, but the risks are not great and recovery will take place without too much disability.

How long a period of hospitalization is necessary for prolapse operations?

Approximately ten to twelve days.

Is there any medical treatment for prolapse?

Yes. The insertion of a pessary will help to keep the uterus and cervix in normal position. However, this form of treatment will not bring about a cure and should not be used as a substitute for surgery unless for some reason the patient cannot undergo an operative procedure.

Why isn't the use of a pessary prolonged indefinitely?

   a. It does not cure the underlying deficiency.

   b. It may lead to an ulceration of the vagina, an inflammation of the vaginal wall, or secondary infection.

   c. The wearing of a pessary requires daily douching.

   d. A pessary requires monthly visits to the doctor's office for removal, cleansing, and replacement.

What is a cystocele?

It is a hernia of the bladder wall into the vagina. Cystoceles may vary in degree from a mild bulge into the vagina to a maximum descent in which almost the entire bladder protrudes through the vaginal opening.

Cystocele. Due to stresses and strains, often occurring during childbirth, a tear of the muscles and ligaments which support the urinary bladder may take place and may result in a hernia of the bladder down toward the vagina. Loss of bladder control may follow, and when this happens, surgical repair should be undertaken.

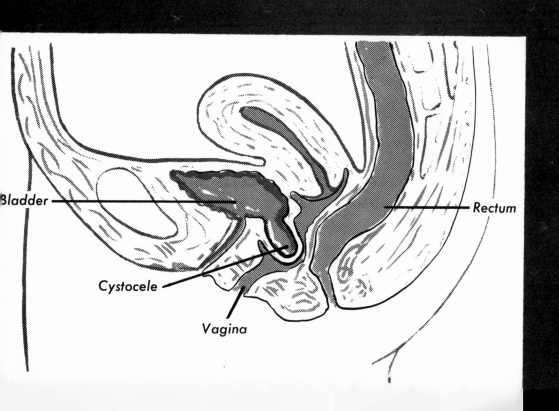

Bladder —   Rectum

Cystocele

Vagina

What is a rectocele?

It is a hernia of the rectal wall into the vagina. Again, the degree of herniation varies markedly from case to case.

What causes cystoceles or rectoceles?

They are caused by the same type of injury that causes a prolapse, that is, a tear of supporting ligaments as a result of childbirth.

How often do cystocele, rectocele, and prolapse occur?

These are common conditions. The incidence is greater in women who have had many children. Also, women past forty are more likely to develop these conditions as their supporting ligaments begin to weaken and stretch.

Rectocele. When the tear in the supporting muscles and ligaments takes place in the posterior portion of the vagina, the rectum may protrude into the vagina. A rectocele is often accompanied by symptoms of marked constipation. Fortunately, this condition too can be repaired readily by surgery.

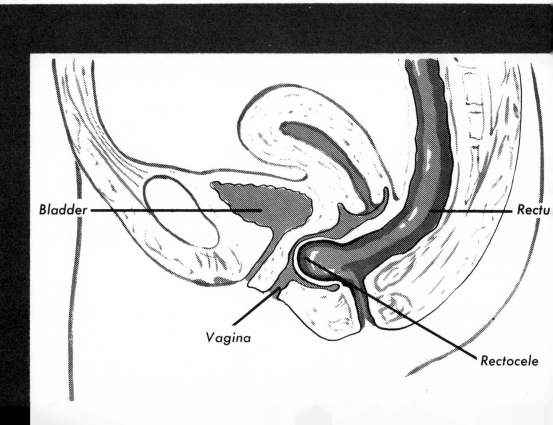

Bladder   Rectu

Vagina

Rectocele

Do cystocele, rectocele, and prolapse tend to occur together?

Yes, in a great number of instances. However, it is entirely possible to have a prolapse without a cystocele or rectocele, or to have a cystocele without a rectocele, or vice versa.

What are the symptoms of cystocele?

The most common symptoms are frequency of urination, loss of urine on coughing, sneezing, laughing, or physical exertion. There may also be a sensation of a bulge into the vagina.

What are the symptoms of rectocele?

A feeling of pressure in the vagina and rectum, with difficulty in evacuating the bowels.

Does cystocele or rectocele and prolapse ever lead to cancer?

No.

What is the treatment for cystocele and rectocele?

A vaginal plastic operation, in which the torn ligaments and muscles are repaired and stretched or excess tissues are excised.

Are operations for cystocele and rectocele serious?

No, but they demand the attention of an expert gynecologist who understands the anatomy and function of the region.

How long a period of hospitalization is necessary following vaginal plastic operations?

One week to ten days.

Are the results of operations for cystocele, rectocele, and prolapse satisfactory?

Yes. Cure can be accomplished in almost all cases.

Can cystocele, rectocele, or prolapse be corrected medically?

No, but temporary relief can be obtained with the use of rings or pessaries. Such appliances do not bring about a cure.

When is surgery necessary for cystocele, rectocele, or prolapse?

When the symptoms, as mentioned previously, are sufficient to interfere with normal happy living, or when bladder or bowel function becomes impaired.

What are the chances of recurrence after surgery?

After competent surgery, the chances of recurrence are less than 5 per cent.

Are there any visible scars following vaginal plastic operations?

No.

What type of anesthesia is used for these procedures?

Either spinal or general anesthesia.

How long do these operations take to perform?

A complete vaginal plastic operation may take anywhere from one to two hours.

Are private nurses necessary after these operations?

Not usually, although they are a great comfort if the patient is able to afford them for a few days.

Are operations upon the vagina very painful?

No.

How soon after vaginal operations is the patient permitted to get out of bed?

On the day following surgery.

Are any special postoperative precautions necessary?

Yes, a catheter may be placed in the bladder for a few days in order to aid restoration of bladder function.

What is the effect of vaginal plastic operations upon the bladder and rectum?

Occasionally, for the first week or two there may be difficulty in urinating. Also, in operations for rectocele there may be difficulty in moving one's bowels for a similar period. These complications are temporary and will subside spontaneously.

Do stitches have to be removed after these operations?

No. The stitches are absorbable and do not have to be removed.

Is it common to bleed after operations upon the vagina?

Yes. Slight staining may continue on and off for several weeks.

Do vaginal plastic operations interfere with marital relations?

No. When the tissues have healed, intercourse can be resumed. This usually takes six to eight weeks.

Can women have babies after surgery for a cystocele or rectocele?

Yes, but delivery may have to be performed by Cesarean section, as surgery may have interfered with the ability of these structures to stretch and dilate sufficiently. Also, vaginal delivery might bring on a recurrence of the cystocele or rectocele.

Can pregnancy take place after surgery for prolapse of the uterus?

Yes, if only the cervix has been removed. Here, too, delivery should be by Cesarean section. Of course, if a hysterectomy has been performed in order to cure the prolapse, pregnancy cannot take place.

When is it best to undergo plastic repair?

After one has completed having children.

How soon after a vaginal plastic operation can one do the following:

Shower	One week.
Bathe	Four weeks.
Walk in the street	One week.
Perform household duties	Two weeks.
Drive a car	Four weeks.
Resume marital relations	Eight weeks.
Return to work	Six weeks.
Douche	Six weeks.

445

What is vaginitis?

It is an inflammation of the vagina.

What causes vaginitis?

a. Gonorrhea.

b. Parasitic infections such as trichomonas.

c. Fungi, such as monilia.

d. Common bacterial infections with staphylococcus, streptococcus, etc.

e. Changes due to old age (senile vaginitis).

f. As a complication of the administration of antibiotic drugs which destroy certain useful vaginal bacteria, vaginitis is occasionally encountered.

Does the healthy vagina contain bacteria?

Yes, and most of these bacteria are beneficial and are not the cause of disease.

What causes parasitic or fungus infections of the vagina?

A change in vaginal acidity which permits these organisms to outgrow the other organisms that are normally present.

What lessens acidity of the vagina?

Menstrual blood will often lessen the acidity and allow harmful organisms to grow and multiply and produce the symptoms of vaginitis.

What are the symptoms of vaginitis?

This will depend upon the cause of the infection. The symptoms of gonorrheal vaginitis will be discussed under the general heading of that disease. Parasitic, fungus, or bacterial vaginitis usually produces the following symptoms:

a. Itching of the vulva.

b. Vaginal discharge.

c. Pain on intercourse.

d. Pain and frequency of urination.

e. Swelling of the external genital structures.

What are the symptoms of senile vaginitis?

Itching, but very little vaginal discharge. There is also pain on intercourse and, rarely, vaginal bleeding.

What tests are performed to determine the type of vaginitis which is present?

A smear of the vaginal discharge is taken and is submitted to microscopic examination. This will demonstrate whether the infection is caused by gonorrhea, monilia, trichomonas, or other bacteria.

What is the treatment for vaginitis?

This will depend upon its cause:

a. Fungus infections are treated successfully with various fungicidal medications. This is usually combined with acid douches.

b. Bacterial vaginitis is treated with the antibiotic drugs, both orally and locally.

c. Senile vaginitis is treated by simple douches and by the administration of female hormones which are applied locally or given generally.

Is there a tendency for vaginitis to recur?

Yes. Many types of vaginitis do have this tendency. For this reason, treatment must be continued over a prolonged period of time. It is common for people to discontinue treatment too quickly because of early relief of symptoms.

What is the most common time for a vaginitis to recur?

After a menstrual period.

Is vaginitis contagious?

Gonorrhea is highly contagious. In rare instances, the trichomonas and monilia can be transferred to the male urethra.

Does vaginitis ever occur in children?

Yes, vulvo-vaginitis is not uncommon in young girls from two to fifteen years of age. The infection is transmitted by poor hygiene and poor toilet habits.

447

Is vulvo-vaginitis in children ever caused by gonorrhea?

Yes. This occasionally happens in homes where sanitary methods are not observed.

What are the symptoms of vaginitis in children?

The child will complain of pain and itching in the region of the vulva. There will also be pain on urination and the parent will notice a vaginal discharge.

What is the treatment for vaginitis in children?

Specific medications should be given for the specific infection. The antibiotics are used to control gonorrhea and most other bacterial infections. Instructions must also be given to improve personal hygiene.

What causes gonorrhea in women?

In almost every instance, it is caused by sexual intercourse with an infected male. Very rarely, gonorrhea may be transmitted from contaminated fingers or bathroom equipment.

What structures in the female genitals are affected by gonorrhea?

The vulva, Bartholin glands, the urethra, the vagina, and the cervix of the uterus are almost always involved in the infection. If the infection extends, it goes up through the cervix into the uterus, out into the Fallopian tubes to the ovaries, and finally to the abdominal cavity, where it causes gonorrheal peritonitis.

What are the symptoms of gonorrhea in the female?

The first symptoms are slight discomfort in the vagina, vaginal discharge, burning, and frequency of urination. These symptoms progress and become more marked for the first few days of the disease.

How is the diagnosis of gonorrhea made?

Microscopic examination reveals the specific causative germ, the gonococcus. *A definite diagnosis is never made unless the actual germ can be seen under the microscope.*

What is the treatment for gonorrhea in the female?

The advent of the sulfa and antibiotic drugs has led to remarkable advancement in the treatment of this disease. *If treated promptly, all the harmful, permanent effects of gonorrhea can be avoided.* All too often, the shame of having a social disease restrains young women from seeking treatment early. The result is that the harmful results have taken too firm a hold before active treatment is instituted. If this has happened, infection of the tubes, ovaries, and abdominal cavity cannot be obliterated completely even with the use of the sulfa or antibiotic drugs.

Does complete recovery take place if treatment for gonorrhea is carried out promptly and adequately?

Yes.

Does gonorrhea interfere with childbearing?

Untreated gonorrhea, or chronic gonorrhea which has affected the tubes and ovaries, will definitely be a factor in the causation of sterility. There is a very high incidence of sterility in women with chronic gonorrhea.

Does gonorrhea ever require surgical treatment?

Yes, under the following conditions:
a. When the Bartholin glands are involved, they may have to be incised or removed.
b. When the Fallopian tubes or ovaries are chronically infected, they may have to be removed.

How does syphilis affect the female genital organs?

A chancre (syphilitic sore) may appear anywhere in the vulva or vagina.

How is the diagnosis of syphilis made in a female?

It is diagnosed by direct examination of a suspicious lesion. A scraping from the sore is taken and is examined under a microscope. The diagnosis is then further confirmed by taking a blood test (Wassermann test, Kahn test, etc.).

What is the usual method of transmission of syphilis?

Through sexual intercourse with an infected male.

What is the treatment for syphilis?

(See Chapter 71, on Venereal Disease.)

Can syphilis interfere with childbearing?

If the syphilis has been treated adequately and promptly, cure can be brought about so that childbearing will probably not be affected. Many investigators used to feel that early miscarriage, premature births, and stillbirths were caused by syphilis. However, with better treatment measures today, this does not occur often.

THE CERVIX

What is the cervix?

The cervix, or neck of the womb, is that portion of the uterus which appears in the vagina. It is a small, firm, muscular organ with a canal through its center (the cervical canal), extending from the vagina to the interior of the body of the uterus. The cervix is the only portion of the uterus that can actually be seen during the course of an office pelvic examination.

How is the cervix examined?

A special instrument known as a speculum is inserted into the vagina.

What is the function of the cervix?

a. It guards the cavity of the uterus from invasion by bacteria or other foreign particles.
b. It allows for the passage of sperm into the cavity of the uterus.
c. It protects the developing embryo during pregnancy.
d. It opens during labor to allow for the passage of the baby.

What is cervicitis?

It is an inflammation of the cervix.

What are the various types of cervicitis?

a. Erosion of the cervix; a raw, reddened area appearing at the opening of the cervical canal in the vagina. This may be primary, appearing in young girls who have a developmental disorder causing an absence of the normal membrane covering of the cervix. Erosions may be secondary, developing as a consequence of injury received during labor, or as a result of operative disturbance, such as after dilatation and curettage.

b. Cystic cervicitis; a condition in which small cysts develop on an inflamed cervix during the healing process. As the surface of the cervix heals, some of its glands are sealed over and form cysts.

c. Hypertrophic cervicitis; a condition in which there is a large overgrowth of the entire substance of the cervical body. It is often associated with cyst formation and erosion.

d. Chronic cervicitis; recurrences of any of the above.

What are the causes of cervicitis?

a. Bacteria, fungi, or parasites.

b. Injury secondary to delivery or surgery.

c. A congenital deficiency in the normal covering layer of the cervix.

What are the symptoms of cervicitis?

a. The most pronounced symptom is vaginal discharge (leukorrhea). The appearance of the discharge may vary from a colorless mucus to a whitish or yellowish discharge.

b. Vaginal bleeding after sexual intercourse.

c. In severe cases, menstrual bleeding may be heavier than normal or may be preceded or followed by staining for a day or two.

Does cervicitis ever interfere with the ability to become pregnant?

Occasionally. In such cases it is necessary to clear up the cervicitis before pregnancy can take place.

What is the treatment for cervicitis?

a. If an infection is present, it must be eradicated by appropriate, specific medication.

b. Douching helps to keep local infection under control; an acid douche may prevent the recurrence of an infection caused by a fungus or parasite.

    c. Simple erosion of a cervix can be treated by cauterizing with silver nitrate applications or by electro-cauterization.

    d. Extensive erosions or cyst formation requires more active and forceful treatment with electro-cauterization.

    e. Chronic hypertrophy of the cervix may be treated by cauterization but the more pronounced cases may require hospitalization for amputation of the cervix.

How is electro-cauterization of the cervix performed?

It is an office procedure in which incisions are burned into the cervix by means of an electrically heated, metal-tipped instrument. The burning incisions, of which many are made, cause the eroded or infected tissue to die and fall away from the underlying healthy cervical tissue. In time, the healthy tissue is able to grow again and to cover the entire cervix.

Is cauterization of the cervix a painful procedure?

No. It is accompanied by relatively little discomfort. There may be a feeling of warmth in the vagina and some cramps may follow, but it does not produce any disability.

How long does cauterization take to perform?

In the hands of a competent gynecologist, only a few minutes.

What is the patient to expect after cauterization of the cervix?

In most instances, there will be an increased vaginal discharge for a week to ten days. This may be heavy, foul-smelling, and grayish in color. After seven or eight days, vaginal bleeding may ensue. This is due to the "sloughing" of the infected tissue.

What precautions should be taken after cauterization of the cervix?

The patient should abstain from intercourse and douches for twelve to fourteen days.

Is it necessary to take douches at any time following cauterization?

Yes. After the slough has been expelled, in about twelve to fourteen days, daily douches with warm water and an acid solution are taken to prevent reinfection. These douches should be continued for approximately three weeks except during the menstrual period.

How long does it take for healing to be complete after cauterization?

Approximately six weeks.

Are medications inserted into the vagina following cauterization?

Some gynecologists recommend the daily insertion of antibiotic vaginal suppositories to prevent reinfection.

Is there a tendency for cervicitis or cervical erosion to recur?

Yes. If it recurs, treatment should be started again. It is not unusual for a slight recurrence to take place, but this will respond if treated promptly.

If cervicitis recurs, should the gynecologist suspect the possibility of a tumor?

Yes, and in such cases a biopsy of the cervical tissue is taken for microscopic examination.

Does the gynecologist examine for cancer in all cases in which there is an abnormality of the cervix?

Yes. A competent gynecologist will be able to decide what type of condition requires further investigation. If there is any doubt as to diagnosis, he will take a cancer smear and do a biopsy of the suspicious area.

What is a cancer smear (Papanicolaou smear)?

It is a method of collecting surface cells from the vagina and cervix and examining them, with special staining techniques, for cancer. It concerns itself with examining those very superficial surface cells which are thrown off (desquamated).

What is the value of the cancer smear?

It can reveal cancer cells at a *very early stage* of their development, thus allowing for extremely early treatment.

Should all women have a cervical cancer smear?

All adult women should have a routine vaginal smear taken every year. Also, a smear should be taken at any time when a lesion is suspected.

Is it painful to take a cancer smear?

Absolutely not. The entire procedure takes no more than a few seconds and is performed merely by swabbing the surface of the cervix and the vagina.

What is a cervical polyp?

It is a small benign tumor arising from the cervix. It usually has a thin stalk and assumes the size and shape of a pea, cherry, or grape.

What causes cervical polyps to grow?

The cause is unknown. They can occur in both young and old women.

Cancer Smear. This is an actual photomicrograph of a Papanicolaou smear. The cells have been taken from the cervix merely by placing a swab into the vaginal orifice. The cells seen in this photograph are all normal.

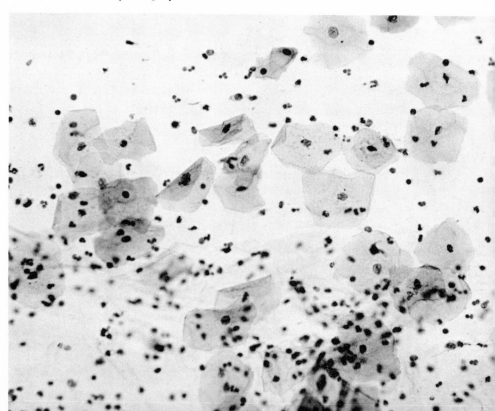

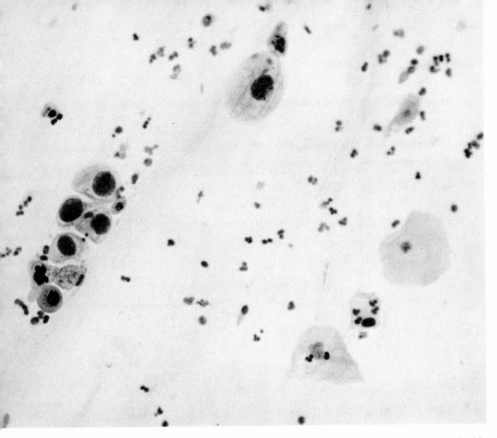

Cancer Smear. In this photomicrograph of a Papanicolaou smear, the very darkly stained cells are cancer cells which have been extruded from the surface of the cervix. Such findings often enable the surgeon to make the diagnosis of cancer in its very earliest stage, thus increasing the chances for cure of this form of cancer. All women past the age of forty should have a Papanicolaou smear taken every year or two.

What are the symptoms of cervical polyps?

Vaginal discharge, staining between periods, pre- and post-menstrual staining, and cramps. One, or all, of these symptoms may appear, or there may be no symptoms whatever.

What is the treatment for cervical polyps?

They should be removed in the office of the gynecologist or, under certain circumstances, in the hospital. This is considered a minor operative procedure and is accompanied by little discomfort.

Do polyps tend to recur?

Once a polyp has been removed it will not regrow. However, women who have developed one polyp do have a tendency to form others. These, too, should be removed.

Are polyps of the cervix ever malignant?

Rarely.

Do polyps interfere with pregnancy?

Usually not.

What is hypertrophy of the cervix?

An overgrowth or elongation of the cervix occurring with or without inflammation. In many cases it is associated with prolapse of the uterus, cystocele, or rectocele. (See section on the External Genitals in this chapter.)

What causes hypertrophy of the cervix?

The cause is unknown.

What are the symptoms of hypertrophy of the cervix?

If it is associated with cystocele, rectocele, or prolapse of the uterus, the symptoms are urinary or rectal. If it exists alone, the symptoms may consist of pressure in the vagina or the presence of a mass protruding through the vaginal opening.

Does hypertrophy of the cervix interfere with marital relations?

Yes. The presence of a mass filling the vagina may make intercourse almost impossible. Pain during intercourse may be the result of displacement of the enlarged cervix.

What is the treatment for hypertrophy of the cervix?

When associated with prolapse, cystocele, or rectocele, the cervix is removed as part of the vaginal plastic operation. When the hypertrophy of the cervix exists alone, it is amputated surgically.

Is amputation of the cervix a major operation?

No. It is considered a minor operation and is accompanied by very little risk or postoperative discomfort.

Where is the incision made for amputation of the cervix?

Entirely within the vaginal canal.

How long a hospital stay is necessary for amputation of the cervix?

Approximately five to six days.

What postoperative precautions are necessary after amputation of the cervix?

It takes approximately three to four weeks to complete convalescence. Marital relations and douching are not permitted for approximately six weeks.

Will amputation of the cervix interfere with subsequent pregnancy?

Pregnancy *can* take place after amputation of the cervix, but delivery will probably be performed by Cesarean section. When the cervix has been amputated, it is often difficult for the neck of the womb to dilate sufficiently to allow for the passage of the baby. Also, there is danger of rupture of this lower segment during labor.

Does hypertrophy of the cervix ever lead to cancer?

No.

Is cancer of the cervix a common condition?

Yes, it accounts for 25 per cent of all cancer found in women!

What causes cancer of the cervix?

The exact cause is unknown. There are many theories, but none of them has been fully substantiated.

At what age is cancer of the cervix usually encountered?

It can occur at any age, but is seen most often in women between forty and sixty years.

Does cancer of the cervix tend to run in families?

No.

Do Jewish women seem to have a certain type of immunity to cancer of the cervix?

It is true that cancer of the cervix is found much less frequently among Jewish women. The exact cause for this odd phenomenon is not known.

457

Is it wise to seek early treatment for any abnormal condition of the cervix in an attempt to prevent cancer?

Definitely, yes. Many competent gynecologists feel that erosion, laceration, inflammation, or benign growths of the cervix may predispose toward cancer formation.

Can cancer of the cervix be prevented?

Cancer prevention is not actually possible, but a *late cancer* can be avoided through early treatment. Thus, periodic vaginal examinations will uncover many cancers in their early curable stages.

What are the early symptoms of cancer of the cervix?

Very early cancer may cause no symptoms whatever. This is one of the main reasons for periodic vaginal examinations. Later on, there may be vaginal discharge, bleeding after intercourse, bleeding after douching, or unexplained bleeding between periods.

Can early cancer of the cervix be detected by a cancer smear?

Yes.

What is non-invasive cancer of the cervix?

This is a condition, also called *in situ* cancer of the cervix, in which the cancer is limited to the most superficial layer of cells and there is no spread to the deeper tissues. This term is used to distinguish it from invasive cancer, in which the spread has extended beyond the superficial layers of cells into the deeper tissues, including the lymph channels and the bloodstream.

How accurate is the cancer smear in diagnosing cancer?

A positive cancer smear is accurate in about 97 per cent of cases.

Does a positive cancer smear constitute sufficient investigation of a cancer of the cervix?

No. Whenever a cancer smear is positive, a biopsy and curettage should be taken to make the diagnosis and location absolutely certain. A positive smear may indicate cancer of the uterine body as well as cancer of the cervix.

What is the treatment for cancer of the cervix?

This will depend entirely upon the stage of development of the cancer at the time it is discovered. There are three ways of treating this disease:

a. By the use of radium and x-ray.
b. By wide surgical removal of the cervix, uterus, tubes, ovaries, and all the lymph channels draining the area.
c. By a combination of radium, x-ray, and surgery.

Who will determine what form of treatment should be administered?

The gynecologist will know which form of treatment to institute after the invasiveness and extent of the cancer have been determined.

What are the chances of recovery from cancer of the cervix?

Early cancer of the cervix can be cured in almost all cases—by either radium, x-ray, surgery, or a combination of these forms of treatment. As the extensiveness of the disease increases and the operative procedures become more involved, recovery rates are lower. In the most extensive cases, the mortality rate is high and the rate of cure is extremely low.

Is it painful to insert radium into the vagina?

No. This procedure is carried out in the hospital, under anesthesia.

Does radium remain inside the body permanently?

No. The radium is usually applied in capsules, and after a sufficient number of radioactive rays have been transmitted, the capsule is removed.

How long does radium usually remain within the genital tract?

Anywhere from 72 to 110 hours, according to the specific dosage indicated.

How long a hospital stay is necessary when radium is inserted?

Anywhere from four to six days.

Is the application of radium followed by postoperative discomfort?

Yes, because extensive packing is inserted into the vagina when radium is being used. This is controlled by use of sedatives.

Is x-ray treatment often given along with radium treatment?

Yes. This is given in the weeks before and after radium implantation, in order to reach parts not reached by the radium.

Are there any postoperative symptoms following radium implantation?

Yes. Disturbance in bowel function and burning and frequency of urination are quite often complications of radium treatment of the cervix.

Does cancer ever recur after radium treatment for cancer of the cervix?

Yes. Some cancers are resistant to radium or inaccessible to it. Recurrence will depend upon the stage of the disease at the time radium and x-ray treatment were given.

Can a patient return to normal living after radium treatment for cancer of the cervix?

Yes, in the majority of instances.

Can a patient become pregnant after radium treatment for cancer of the cervix?

Because ovarian function will have been destroyed by the radium treatment, pregnancy will not take place. Menstruation will also cease as a result of radium therapy.

What type of surgery is performed for cancer of the cervix?

a. Radical hysterectomy for *in situ* or early invasive cancer.
b. Exenteration for extensive and advanced cancer.

What is meant by an exenteration operation for cancer of the cervix?

This is an extremely complicated operative procedure in which the entire uterus, cervix, vagina, tubes, ovaries, lymph glands, bladder, and/or rectum are removed for extensive cancer. Artificial openings are made for the passage of urine and stool.

Can cancer of the cervix be cured by such radical surgery?

Only the occasional case. It must be remembered that this type of surgery is carried out only on those who have extensive cancer and who would have died without surgery.

Is this operation dangerous?

Yes.

What is the future outlook for those afflicted with cancer of the cervix?

Earlier detection can lead to a substantially higher cure rate in years to come. The advent of the cancer smear now permits the diagnosis to be made at earlier stages in the development of the disease.

THE UTERUS

What is the uterus?

The uterus, or womb, is a pear-shaped muscular organ lying in the middle of the pelvis. It is approximately three inches long, two inches wide, and one inch thick. It consists of an outer, smooth covering, a middle layer composed of thick muscle tissue, and an inner cavity lined with endometrial cells. The cavity of the uterus connects with the vagina through the cervix, and connects with the abdominal cavity through the Fallopian tubes. The hollow Fallopian tubes open within the abdominal cavity near the ovaries. The uterus is supported and suspended by several ligaments.

What is the exact position of the uterus?

It lies just above the pubic bones, behind the urinary bladder, in front of the rectum and above the vagina.

What are the functions of the uterus?

a. To prepare for the reception of a fertilized egg.
b. To nurture and harbor the embryo during its development.
c. To expel the baby when it is mature and ready for delivery.

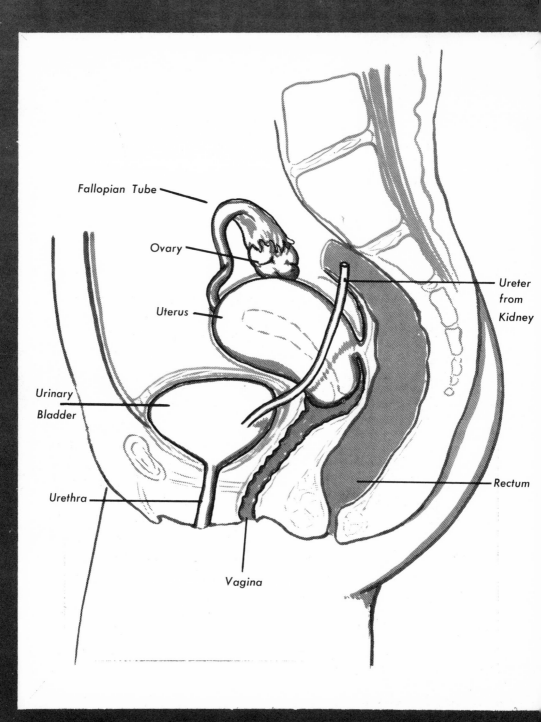

Fallopian Tube

Ovary

Uterus

Ureter from Kidney

Urinary Bladder

Urethra

Rectum

Vagina

The Female Organs. This diagram shows the female reproductive organs: the uterus, the fallopian tubes, and the ovaries. Note the relation of the female reproductive organs to surrounding structures in the pelvic region.

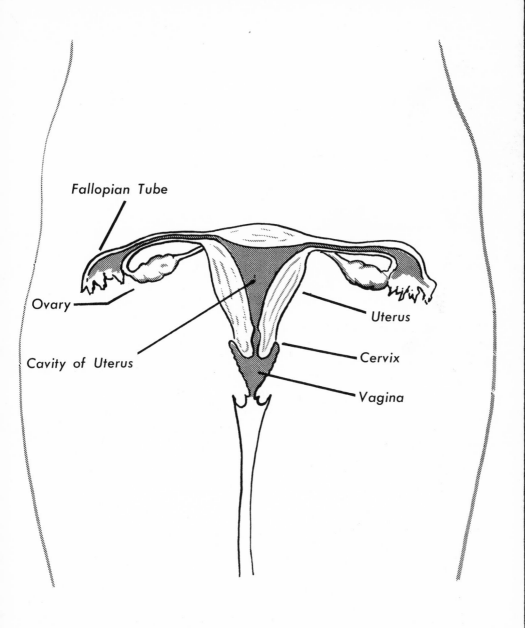

Fallopian Tube

Ovary

Cavity of Uterus

Uterus

Cervix

Vagina

The Female Organs. This frontal diagram of the female reproductive organs gives another view of these anatomical structures. Young people today should be made famil-iar with the normal structure of their own bodies so that they can better understand

What influences the uterus to prepare for pregnancy?

Hormones which are secreted by the ovaries and the other endocrine glands. If the fertilized egg is not forthcoming, menstruation ensues and the uterine lining is shed. This process is repeated each month, from puberty to menopause, unless there is a glandular upset or, of course, unless pregnancy exists.

What is the significance of a tipped womb?

Ordinarily, this condition has no significance.

What symptoms are caused by a tipped womb?

Usually none. In rare instances, backache and a dragging sensation in the lower pelvic region may occur with the finding of a womb that is tipped markedly in a backward direction.

What is the treatment for a tipped womb?

The great majority of cases require no treatment whatever. (The large number of operations for "straightening out" the womb, which were performed years ago, have now been abandoned as unnecessary operative procedures.) In rare instances, a vaginal pessary is employed to maintain a forward position of the uterus.

Does a tipped womb interfere with pregnancy?

Definitely not.

Does a tipped womb interfere with intercourse?

No.

What is an infantile uterus?

This is a term formerly used to describe a small-sized uterus.

What is the significance of an infantile uterus?

None, providing the uterus functions normally. In other words, if menstruation is normal and pregnancy can take place, a small-sized uterus is of no significance.

Do women with an infantile uterus have difficulty in becoming pregnant?

Not if their menstrual function is normal.

What is a curettage?

This is an operation performed upon the cavity of the uterus through the vagina. It consists of scraping out the lining membrane of the uterus. Special instruments are used to dilate the cervix and to scrape out the uterine cavity.

Why is curettage performed?

a. For diagnostic purposes.

b. For therapeutic purposes.

c. A curettage is often diagnostic and therapeutic at the same time, as in cases of hyperplasia or polyps of the uterus.

When is a diagnostic curettage performed?

a. In cases of unexplained uterine bleeding.

b. In cases in which a polyp of the uterine cavity is suspected.

c. In cases in which a cancer of the body of the uterus is suspected.

d. In cases in which tuberculosis of the lining of the uterus is suspected.

When is a therapeutic curettage performed?

a. When a disorder, such as a polyp, of the lining membrane of the uterus has already been diagnosed, curettage may result in a cure.

b. When an overgrowth of the lining membrane of the uterus (endometrial hyperplasia) has been diagnosed, a curettage will often bring about a cure.

c. Following a miscarriage, when parts of the fetus or placenta remain behind. Curettage in such instances will clean out the cavity and thus restore normalcy.

What is another name for curettage?

It is commonly called a "D and C" operation. This stands for dilatation and curettage.

465

Is "D and C" a painful operation?

No. It is performed under general anesthesia in the hospital.

How long a hospital stay is necessary following curettage?

Approximately three days.

Are there any visible incisions following curettage?

No. It is done completely through the vagina.

How soon after this curettage can one return to work?

Within one week.

What restrictions must be followed after curettage?

Douching and intercourse must not be performed for four to six weeks.

Can normal pregnancy take place after a curettage?

Yes. A curettage performed by a competent gynecologist in a hospital will not interfere with subsequent pregnancies.

What is endometritis?

It is an infection of the lining of the uterus.

What causes endometritis?

a. Gonorrhea.

b. It may follow a miscarriage or abortion, particularly after a criminal attempt has been made to induce abortion.

c. It may follow normal delivery where an accidental infection of the uterus has taken place.

d. Tuberculosis, where spread to the uterus has come about secondary to infection in the lungs or kidney.

What are the symptoms of endometritis?

Irregular bleeding, vaginal discharge, pain and tenderness in the lower abdomen, a feeling of weakness, fever, urinary distress, etc.

What is the treatment for endometritis?

The first step is to determine the exact cause. If there has been an incomplete miscarriage, the uterine cavity must be emptied by the performance of a curettage. If the endometritis has been caused by bacterial infection, antibiotic drugs should be given. If the infection has extended beyond the lining membrane into the wall of the uterus, it may be necessary to remove the uterus in order to effect a cure.

Does endometritis ever heal by itself?

Yes, in certain cases. More often, the infection will spread outward to involve the deeper layers of the uterus, the tubes, the ovaries, and even the abdominal cavity.

What is an endometrial polyp?

It is a growth arising from the lining of the uterus and extending into the uterine cavity. Often, there are multiple polyps.

What are the symptoms of an endometrial polyp?

Cramplike menstrual pain, staining between periods, excessive menstrual bleeding, and vaginal discharge.

How is the diagnosis of an endometrial polyp made?

By diagnostic curettage, or by the performance of a hysterogram.

What is a hysterogram?

It is an x-ray investigation of the cavity of the uterus performed by injecting an opaque dye through the cervix into the uterine cavity. When films are taken, they will show the outline of the cavity.

Do endometrial polyps ever become malignant?

Yes, occasionally.

What is the treatment for endometrial polyps?

They are removed by curettage. When they protrude through the cervix into the vaginal canal, they can be removed by clamping or crushing with an instrument through the vagina. If there is any evidence of malignant change within the polyp, a total hysterectomy (complete removal of the uterus and cervix) must be performed.

467

What is endometrial hyperplasia?

It is an overgrowth of the lining of the uterus.

What causes endometrial hyperplasia?

It is usually associated with excessive and prolonged production of female sex hormone (estrogen) by the ovaries. Frequently, an ovarian cyst or tumor is present and may be responsible for the production of excess estrogen.

What are the symptoms of endometrial hyperplasia?

It is characterized by completely irregular and unpredictable bleeding, varying from total lack of menstruation to more frequent periods than normal, and from slight staining to profuse bleeding. Characteristically, endometrial hyperplasia results in painless bleeding.

Does endometrial hyperplasia have anything to do with inability to become pregnant (infertility)?

Yes. Women with endometrial hyperplasia often do not ovulate and therefore cannot become pregnant.

How is endometrial hyperplasia diagnosed?

By microscopic examination of tissue which is taken from the lining of the uterus by endometrial biopsy. Also, by examination of tissue removed by curettage.

Where and how is an endometrial biopsy performed?

This is an office procedure and is performed simply by the insertion of a special instrument through the vagina and cervix into the uterine cavity. A small piece of tissue is removed and is examined microscopically.

Is endometrial biopsy a painful procedure?

No. It is a simple office procedure accompanied by a minimal amount of discomfort.

What is the treatment for endometrial hyperplasia?

This depends upon the age of the patient, the type of hyperplasia found on microscopic examination, and the presence or absence of accompanying ovarian growths. In young females still in the child-bearing age, simple hyperplasia is treated by curettage and by use of estrogen and progesterone (ovarian hormones) to simulate the normal menstrual cycle. This is called cyclic therapy.

After menopause, depending upon the type of hyperplasia, the treatment varies from simple curettage to hysterectomy. If the hyperplasia recurs, or shows a preponderance of certain types of cells, and if the patient is past the childbearing age, hysterectomy will probably be the best treatment. In the presence of an enlarged ovary, hyperplasia must be suspected as being related to a tumor of the ovary. In these cases, an abdominal operation should be performed and the ovaries and uterus removed.

Is there any connection between endometrial hyperplasia and cancer of the uterus?

In women past the childbearing age, it is thought that certain types of endometrial hyperplasia may be associated with development of cancer of the uterus. For this reason, more radical treatment is advised for older women with endometrial hyperplasia.

Should women who have endometrial hyperplasia return for frequent periodic examinations?

Yes. Any irregularity in the menstrual cycle, if a woman is still in the childbearing age, should stimulate a visit to the gynecologist.

What is the treatment of choice for recurrent hyperplasia in young women?

a. Repeated curettage, or cyclic hormone therapy for a prolonged period.

b. If symptoms of hyperplasia cannot be controlled, it may be necessary to perform a hysterectomy even in a young woman. Fortunately, this is rarely necessary.

What is the incidence of cancer of the body of the uterus?

It is the second most common cancer of the female genital tract. However, cancer of the cervix is five times more frequent than cancer of the body of the uterus.

Who is most likely to develop cancer of the uterus?

It occurs at a later age than cancer of the cervix. It is most prevalent in women past fifty.

Is there a tendency to inherit cancer of the uterus?

No.

What is the difference between cancer and sarcoma of the uterus?

Cancer arises from the lining membrane of the uterus, while sarcoma (an equally malignant tumor) arises from the muscle layer of the uterus.

What are the symptoms of cancer of the uterus?

a. Irregular vaginal bleeding in women still having menstrual periods.
b. Bleeding after the menopause.
c. Enlargement of the uterus.

How is cancer of the uterus diagnosed?

By performing diagnostic curettage. Any bleeding in a woman past her menopause must be looked upon with suspicion and must be investigated by curettage to rule out cancer. A cancer smear and an endometrial biopsy are also helpful in establishing the diagnosis.

What treatment is advocated for cancer of the uterus?

Application of radium, followed in four to six weeks by total hysterectomy.

Is this a serious procedure?

Yes, but recovery from the surgery will take place in almost all cases.

What is the rate of cure for cancer of the body of the uterus?

If the cancer is detected before it has extended beyond the confines of the uterus, approximately four out of five cases can be cured. In cases where spread has already gone beyond the uterus, only about one out of eight can be cured.

Is it possible to prevent cancer of the uterus?

It cannot be prevented, but it *can* be detected earlier if women seek medical help as soon as they notice abnormal vaginal bleeding.

What are fibroids (leiomyoma) of the uterus?

Fibroids are benign tumors composed of muscle tissue. They tend to be round in shape and firm in consistency.

What causes fibroids?

Although the exact cause is unknown, it has been found that certain ovarian hormones play an important role in the speed of growth. Thus, after menopause, when very little ovarian hormone is being secreted, fibroids stop growing and may even shrink.

What is the incidence of fibroids?

Almost 25 per cent of all women have fibroids of the uterus. The majority of such growths cause no symptoms and demand no treatment.

When are women most likely to develop fibroids?

During the later stages of the childbearing period, that is, between the ages of forty and fifty years. However, they may be found in women in their early twenties or in those past menopause.

Do fibroids tend to run in families?

There is no actual inherited tendency, but since one in four women have fibroids it is not uncommon to find more than one member of a family with this condition.

What are the various types of fibroids?

a. Subserous; those growing beneath the outer coat of the uterus.
b. Intramural; those growing in the muscular layer of the uterus.
c. Submucous; those growing beneath the lining membrane of the uterine cavity.

Do fibroids vary greatly in size?

Yes. They may be as small as a pinhead or as large as a watermelon. They are almost always multiple.

471

What are the symptoms of fibroids?

a. Many fibroids cause no symptoms and are found inadvertently on routine pelvic examination.
b. If the fibroid is submucous in type, it may cause uterine bleeding between periods or prolonged heavy menstruation.
c. Intramural and subserous fibroids may cause excessive menstrual bleeding but may produce no symptoms at all.
d. There may be frequency of urination and difficulty in bowel function if the fibroids grow to a large size and press upon the bladder or rectum.
e. Backache or lower abdominal pain occurs occasionally.
f. Infertility may ensue if the fibroid distorts the uterine cavity.

How is the diagnosis of fibroids made?

By manual pelvic examination. Such a vaginal examination will reveal the size, shape, and other features of the tumor. A hysterogram may help to diagnose small submucous fibroids.

Is a fibroid of the uterus a malignant tumor?

Definitely not. Fibroids are benign growths!

Do fibroids become cancerous?

No. Occasionally, cancer develops in a uterus containing fibroids, but the presence of the fibroid does not predispose toward the development of the cancer.

Are fibroids found in association with other conditions within the uterus?

Yes. There is a high incidence of endometrial polyps and endometrial hyperplasia in those patients who have fibroids.

What is the best treatment for fibroids?

If the fibroids produce symptoms or grow rapidly, they should be removed surgically.

What operative procedures are performed for fibroids?

When only the fibroids are removed, it is called a myomectomy. When the entire uterus is removed, it is termed a hysterectomy.

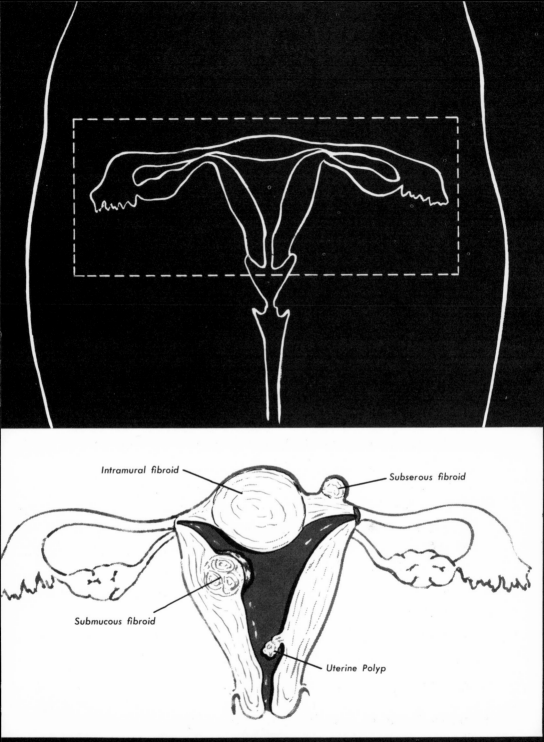

Intramural fibroid

Subserous fibroid

Submucous fibroid

Uterine Polyp

Fibroids of the Uterus. This diagram shows various forms of fibroid tumors of the uterus and where they are located. These tumors are not malignant but can cause serious symptoms, such as bleeding between menstrual periods or, if they grow large enough, pressure upon the urinary bladder or rectum. When symptoms are pronounced or when the tumors grow very large, the surgeon may recommend their removal.

How does a gynecologist decide whether to do a myomectomy or a hysterectomy?

This will depend upon the *age* of the patient and her desire to have children. If the patient desires children, an attempt will be made to preserve the uterus and a myomectomy will be performed.

Are there methods of treating fibroids other than myomectomy or hysterectomy?

Yes. Some small submucous fibroids can be removed by simple curettage, when they develop into polyp-like growths.

Do fibroids have a tendency to recur?

Ten per cent will recur following myomectomy. Of course, if the entire uterus is removed, fibroids cannot recur.

Must all fibroids be operated upon?

No. A fair proportion require no treatment whatever.

What are the indications for surgical removal of fibroids?

a. Increased, prolonged, and more frequent menstruation.
b. Episodes of severe bleeding between periods.
c. Pressure symptoms causing continued urinary or rectal discomfort.
d. Rapid increase in the size of a fibroid.
e. Any fibroid larger than the size of a three months' pregnancy should be removed even if it causes no symptoms.
f. Acute pain due to degeneration of a fibroid or to a twist in a fibroid.
g. Repeated miscarriage or sterility.

Do fibroids ever occur during pregnancy?

Yes. When present, they may increase in size as the pregnancy grows.

Should a fibroid be treated during pregnancy?

No. It is best to postpone treatment until after the baby is born.

Can a woman become pregnant after surgery for fibroids?

If a myomectomy has been performed, subsequent pregnancy is possible. In such cases, the baby may have to be delivered by Cesarean section.

Is the surgical treatment of fibroids usually successful?

Yes, a cure is the result in almost all cases.

Is there any treatment for fibroids of the uterus other than surgery?

a. Yes. Temporary relief may be obtained in some cases by the administration of male sex hormones. This may stop the heavy vaginal flow, but it will not reduce the size of a fibroid.

b. X-ray therapy has been used for the smaller fibroids, but it is not considered a satisfactory form of treatment.

Is myomectomy considered a major operation?

Yes, since it involves an abdominal incision. However, recovery takes place in almost all instances. Hospitalization for ten to twelve days is usually required.

Does menstruation return to normal after myomectomy?

Yes.

How long does it take to recover from the effects of myomectomy?

Approximately six weeks.

How long should a woman wait after myomectomy before attempting pregnancy?

Nine to twelve months.

What is hysterectomy?

An operation for the removal of the uterus.

What are the various types of hysterectomy?

a. Subtotal or supracervical hysterectomy; removal of the body of the uterus leaving the cervix behind.

b. Total hysterectomy; removal of the body of the uterus and the cervix.

c. Radical hysterectomy; this includes removal of a good portion of

475

the vagina, the tubes and ovaries, the supporting tissues and lymph glands along with the body and cervix of the uterus.

d. Porro section; removal of the uterus at the time of delivery of a baby by Cesarean section.

e. Vaginal hysterectomy; removal of the uterus and cervix through the vagina instead of through an abdominal incision.

What are some of the indications for hysterectomy?

a. Symptomatic fibroids.
b. Chronic, incurable inflammatory disease of the uterus, tubes, and ovaries, such as gonorrhea or tuberculosis.
c. Severe recurrent endometrial hyperplasia.
d. Cancer of the uterus or cervix.
e. Cancer of the tubes or ovaries.
f. Chronic disabling endometriosis.
g. Uncontrollable hemorrhage following delivery of a baby.
h. In certain cases where the ovaries must be removed for cysts or growths, the uterus should also be removed.
i. Rupture of the uterus during pregnancy.

Is hysterectomy a major operative procedure?

Yes. However, it is not considered a dangerous operation, and operative recovery occurs in almost 100 per cent of the cases.

Does a woman menstruate after hysterectomy?

No.

Can a patient become pregnant after hysterectomy?

No.

Must the ovaries always be removed when hysterectomy is performed?

If the disease for which the hysterectomy has been performed is cancerous in nature, the tubes and ovaries must be removed. If the condition is benign, and the woman is still under forty years of age, one or both ovaries may be left in place, so that the uncomfortable symptoms of change of life do not ensue. Every attempt is made to leave the ovaries in place when the patient is exceptionally young. They are removed when the patient is more than forty years of age. If the ovaries are inflamed or abscessed, or if endometriosis is present, the ovaries are removed when performing a hysterectomy.

Do ovaries left behind after hysterectomy tend to degenerate and become cystic?

There is no conclusive evidence on this subject, although it has been common medical teaching that this does occur.

Do the symptoms of menopause (change of life) always follow hysterectomy?

No. If one or both ovaries are left behind, menopause will not follow. Menopause occurs only when both ovaries have been removed.

Can the symptoms of menopause be controlled after hysterectomy?

Yes. There are excellent means of combatting the symptoms of menopause.

Does the removal of the uterus affect one's sex life in any way?

No. The removal of the uterus, with or without the removal of the ovaries, does not affect sexual ability or sexual desire. As a matter of fact, some women state that they are happier in their marital relations after hysterectomy than before.

Are the external genitals altered during hysterectomy?

No. The vagina and other external genital structures are unaffected by hysterectomy.

Will hysterectomy cause changes in the physical appearance of a woman?

No. This is a common misconception. Women do *not* tend to become fat or to lose their feminine characteristics because of hysterectomy! It must be remembered, though, that most hysterectomies are performed in the fifth and sixth decades of life, when women ordinarily show signs of aging.

477

Is the scar of hysterectomy disfiguring?

No. It is a simple line on the abdomen. If a vaginal hysterectomy has been performed, no scar will be visible.

What are the indications for the performance of a vaginal hysterectomy?

When there is prolapse of the uterus along with a cystocele and rectocele, it is sometimes advisable to remove the uterus through the vagina so that a vaginal plastic operation can be performed at the same time. This cannot be done if the uterus is enlarged to such an extent that it cannot be delivered through the vagina. Vaginal hysterectomy is not indicated when a malignancy is suspected.

Is vaginal hysterectomy a dangerous operative procedure?

No. It carries with it the same risks as hysterectomy performed through an abdominal incision.

Is hysterectomy a painful operation?

There is the same discomfort that follows any abdominal operation. Most pain can be controlled readily by medication.

How long does it take to perform the average hysterectomy?

From one to two hours.

How soon after hysterectomy can a patient get out of bed?

Usually, the day following the operation.

How long a hospital stay is necessary following hysterectomy?

Nine to twelve days.

What postoperative symptoms follow hysterectomy?

There may be vaginal bleeding or discharge for a week or two. There may also be difficulty in passing urine or in moving the bowels for a week or more after hysterectomy.

How soon after hysterectomy can one do the following:

Bathe	Four weeks.
Walk in the street	Eight to ten days.
Drive a car	Four to five weeks.
Perform all household duties	Eight weeks.
Resume marital relations	Eight weeks.
Return to work	Eight weeks.
Resume all physical activities	Three months.

What is endometriosis?

A condition in which the lining cells of the uterus (endometrial cells) are found in abnormal locations. These cells may be found deep within the wall of the uterus, on the outer coat of the uterus, the Fallopian tubes, the ovaries, the uterine ligaments, bowel, bladder, vagina, or in other places within the abdominal cavity.

How do these endometrial cells exist in abnormal positions?

They implant upon the surface of other structures and grow as small nests of cells. They vary in size from that of a pinhead to the size of an orange. They often form cysts which contain a chocolate-appearing fluid that represents old bloody menstrual-like material.

What abnormal conditions are produced by these endometrial implants?

They may cause firm adhesions between the tubes and the ovaries or the bladder, the bowel or the uterus. They may form cysts. These cysts may twist or rupture, causing acute abdominal pain and distress.

Do these endometrial implants function like normal uterine cells?

Yes. They become distended and engorged with blood as each menstrual period approaches, and they bleed when menstruation takes place.

What causes endometriosis?

The exact cause is unknown. One theory is that the lining cells of the uterus are expelled through the Fallopian tubes by a reverse peristaltic action in the tubes during menstrual periods. Another theory is that these cells are dislodged following surgery upon the uterus.

What are some of the symptoms of endometriosis?

a. It may cause no symptoms whatever and be discovered accidentally at operation for another condition.

b. There may be marked pain before and during the menstrual period.

c. There may be marked pain on urination, defecation, or during intercourse.

d. Menstrual bleeding may be markedly increased.

e. Inability to become pregnant is a complication of extensive endometriosis.

What is the treatment for endometriosis?

a. Treatment is usually medical and will include the administration of male sex hormones or enough female sex hormones to temporarily stop menstrual periods. However, this type of treatment cannot be pursued indefinitely.

b. In persistent cases of endometriosis with marked symptoms, hysterectomy may have to be performed. This is reserved for women past the childbearing age or for those whose symptoms are so severe that they demand treatment.

c. In young women in the childbearing age, pregnancy causes temporary relief, since the cyclic influence which causes the symptoms of endometriosis is interrupted.

Does endometriosis lead to cancer?

No.

What can happen if endometriosis is permitted to go untreated?

The symptoms may become progressive and debilitating. If the endometriosis involves the bowel or intestinal tract, obstruction of the bowel may take place. In certain cases, endometrial cysts will grow so large that they will create pressure on other organs and will demand surgery. Endometrial cysts sometimes twist or rupture, thus requiring immediate surgical intervention.

A B O R T I O N
(*Miscarriage*)

What is an abortion?

It is the expulsion of the products of conception from the uterus during the first six months of the pregnancy. Abortion applies to loss of pregnancy at a time when the fetus is unable to maintain life on its own.

When is the fetus considered to be living or viable?

Not until the twenty-sixth to twenty-eighth week of its development.

Does the term "abortion" always mean that there has been an illegal procedure?

No. Among medical people, abortion refers only to the fact that the pregnancy has ended at a time when the fetus is not yet sufficiently developed to be able to maintain life.

What are the various kinds of abortion?

a. Spontaneous abortion, where no artificial means have been used to bring it on.
b. Induced abortion, where instrumentation, medication, or operation have been used to bring about the termination of the pregnancy.

Are there various types of spontaneous abortion?

Yes. They are:

a. Threatened abortion.
b. Inevitable abortion.
c. Incomplete abortion.
d. Complete abortion.
e. Infected abortion.
f. Missed abortion.

Are there various types of induced abortion?

Yes. They are:

a. Therapeutic or legal abortion.
b. Criminal or illegal abortion.

481

How often does miscarriage or abortion occur?

In this country, about one out of every eight to ten pregnancies terminates in abortion. These include all the types listed above.

What are some of the common causes of spontaneous abortion?

a. Defects in the egg, the sperm, the fertilized egg, or the placenta.
b. Disease of the uterus, such as an infection or a fibroid tumor.
c. Upset in the glandular system associated with ovarian, thyroid, or pituitary dysfunction.
d. Constitutional diseases, such as diabetes, malnutrition, syphilis, tuberculosis, etc.
e. Exposure to excessive x-ray radiation, the taking of poisons, etc.
f. Extreme physical injury or shock.
g. Extreme emotional upset.

What is a threatened abortion?

It is a state during early pregnancy in which there is vaginal staining and abdominal cramps but the cervix remains undilated and the products of conception are not expelled.

What is inevitable abortion?

It is a state in which bleeding and dilatation of the cervix are so advanced that nothing can be done to prevent expulsion of the fetus from the uterus.

What is incomplete abortion?

This refers to a condition in which there has been only partial expulsion of the products of conception.

What is a complete abortion?

It is a state wherein the entire fetal sac and placenta have been fully expelled from the uterus.

What are the symptoms of spontaneous abortion?

a. In the early stages of threatened abortion, staining is the only positive sign. Slight cramps or backache may then develop. This state often continues for days or even weeks.

b. In inevitable abortion, bleeding is heavier, cramps become regular, severe, and progressive, and the cervix begins to dilate.

c. In incomplete abortion, cramps and bleeding are marked, pieces of tissue or clots are passed, and the cervix is dilated.

d. In complete abortion, after increasingly severe cramps and passage of clots, a large mass is expelled from the vagina. On examination, it will be found to contain all the products of conception.

What is the treatment for threatened abortion?

a. Bed rest.

b. Hormone therapy.

c. Administration of vitamins C and K.

d. The giving of sedatives.

Is the treatment of threatened abortion successful?

Not always. Many cases will go on to abortion no matter what treatment is carried out.

What is the treatment for inevitable abortion?

When it is obvious that abortion is inevitable, the uterus should be emptied. The evaluation of the inevitability of an abortion is difficult to make, but all gynecologists will give the patient every opportunity to maintain the pregnancy. When it is obvious that this is impossible, it is best to empty the uterus completely by curettage.

What is the treatment for incomplete abortion?

A curettage should be performed in order to clean out the cavity of the uterus completely. If a great deal of bleeding has been associated with the miscarriage, blood transfusions should be given.

What is the treatment for complete abortion?

No treatment is necessary unless severe blood loss has taken place. In that event, transfusions should be given. If there is evidence of infection, antibiotic drugs should be prescribed.

What is a missed abortion?

This is a state of pregnancy wherein the fetus has died and has been separated from the uterine wall but, instead of being expelled, is retained within the uterine cavity. Missed abortion is a very trying situation for the patient, since the correct treatment must be conservative, thereby permitting the dead embryo to remain within the uterus for periods up to several weeks. In certain cases, medications are given to bring on the onset of labor. However, the safest course is to wait for the uterus to empty itself spontaneously. This may not occur until many weeks after the fetus has lost its viability (ability to live).

What is habitual abortion?

This is a term applied to repeated abortions in the same patient. The signs, symptoms, and treatment are the same for each abortion.

What are thought to be the causes for habitual abortion?

a. Glandular imbalance involving the pituitary, thyroid, or ovaries.
b. Emotional imbalance of a deep and severe nature.
c. Uterine malformation, present since birth.

Can habitual abortion ever be helped by medical treatment?

Yes, but it demands thorough investigation into all its aspects and intensive treatment by the physician.

What percentage of abortions require curettage?

Approximately 50 per cent of spontaneous abortions are complete and require no operative procedure. If there is any doubt, a curettage should be done to forestall further bleeding.

When does abortion require hospitalization?

When the bleeding is profuse or when abdominal cramps become severe and persistent.

What are the greatest dangers associated with abortion?

a. In incomplete abortion, bleeding may be so profuse as to threaten life. In such cases, prompt transfusions are lifesaving.
b. Infection following abortion is a not uncommon complication, especially when performed criminally under unsterile conditions. This will require active, strenuous treatment with the antibiotic drugs.

484

Can infection follow any type of abortion?

Yes, but it is rare when performed legally in a hospital operating room.

What are the consequences of improper treatment of abortion?

a. Infection may set in and may necessitate removal of the uterus, tubes, and ovaries.

b. Sterility may ensue.

What restrictions are imposed following miscarriage?

a. Rest for one to two weeks.

b. No douches or tub baths for one month.

c. No marital relations for one month.

What are the legal indications for therapeutic abortion?

The laws of each state vary markedly in their interpretation of therapeutic abortion. Broadly speaking, most states permit interruption of pregnancy only when the life of the mother is seriously endangered. The evaluation of a specific danger is subject to wide variations of opinion and interpretation.

In many states, severe heart conditions, tuberculosis, serious kidney conditions, and mental illness are considered to be the main indications for the legal interruption of pregnancy.

When should a therapeutic abortion be performed, if at all?

Before the twelfth week of pregnancy. If the pregnancy is to be interrupted at all after the twelfth week, it must be accomplished through the performance of a hysterotomy, a major surgical procedure. This is quite similar to a Cesarean section done at full term and will carry the same risks.

What are the dangers of a criminal abortion?

Illegally induced or criminal abortion is fraught with great danger to the patient. The mortality rate from criminal abortion is extremely high and constitutes a major portion of the maternal deaths that occur. Abortion should never be performed anywhere except in an approved hospital where sterile technique, adequate anesthesia, and

485

equipment for blood transfusion are always available. Fatal hemorrhage, infection, perforation of the uterus, etc., are all too frequent complications of criminal attempts to empty the uterus.

Is the incidence of sterility very great following criminal abortion?

Yes. This is one of the most common causes for inability to become pregnant.

Is it a criminal offense to recommend someone to an abortionist?

Yes. One who recommends a criminal abortion is judged to be almost as guilty as the abortionist himself.

THE FALLOPIAN TUBES
(The Uterine Tubes)

What are the Fallopian tubes?

They are two hollow, tubelike structures which arise at the upper end of the borders of the uterus and extend outward to each side of the pelvis for a distance of three to four inches. Each tube is the width of a lead pencil and at its most distant point is funnel-shaped. The tubes are composed of an outer layer of muscle and an inner lining membrane covered with hairlike projections. These projections have a swaying, sweeping motion which helps to send the egg down toward the uterus and may aid the sperm in coming up through the tube to reach the egg.

What is the function of the Fallopian tubes?

To transport the egg which has been discharged from the ovary down to the uterine cavity. To permit sperm to pass from the uterine cavity up toward the egg.

What is salpingitis?

A bacterial infection of the Fallopian tubes.

What are the most common causes of infection within the Fallopian tubes?

a. Gonorrhea, which has ascended via the vagina, cervix, and uterus.

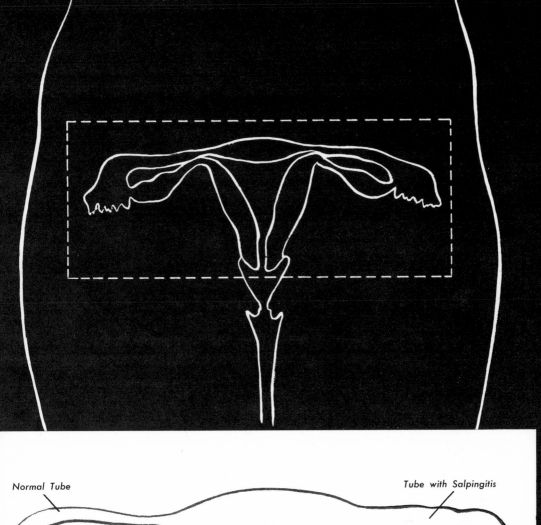

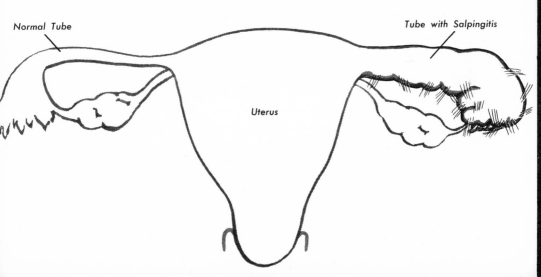

Normal Tube

Tube with Salpingitis

Uterus

Salpingitis. This diagram shows an inflammation of a fallopian tube, a condition often caused by untreated gonorrhea. Salpingitis is one of the greatest causes of sterility in women. Prompt treatment of gonorrhea will prevent most cases of salpingitis.

b. Tuberculosis, usually secondary to a primary infection elsewhere.

c. Staphylococcus, pneumococcus, or streptococcus infections.

Is salpingitis a common condition?

Yes, but with the advent of the antibiotic drugs and the discovery of medications to control tuberculosis, inflammation of the tubes is much less frequently encountered than it was ten, twenty, or more years ago.

What harm may result from an infection within the Fallopian tubes?

a. Sterility.

b. Tubal pregnancy (ectopic pregnancy).

c. The formation of a chronic abscess involving the ovary as well as the tube.

d. Spread of the infection out into the abdominal cavity, thus causing peritonitis.

What treatment must often be instituted in order to cure chronic infection of the Fallopian tubes?

Surgery, with removal of the uterus, tubes, and ovaries.

What are the symptoms of acute salpingitis?

Lower abdominal pain, fever, chills, difficulty on urination, nausea and vomiting, vaginal discharge, increased menstrual bleeding, vaginal bleeding between periods, pain on intercourse, etc. Some, or all, of these symptoms may be encountered in salpingitis.

What is the best way to prevent salpingitis?

Of course, women should avoid relations with infected men. However, whenever vaginal discharge develops following intercourse, it should be treated promptly by a gynecologist. This can, in the great majority of cases, prevent the spread of the infection through the uterus into the Fallopian tubes.

What is the treatment for salpingitis once it has developed?

Acute salpingitis is treated with the antibiotic drugs. The patient is put to bed and given medications to relieve pain. If an abscess has formed and it persists, surgery, with removal of the tube, may be necessary.

Is surgery usually performed during the acute phase of salpingitis?

No. The gynecologist will make every attempt to bring the inflammation under control by medical means. Immediate surgery may be necessary when an abscess within the tube is threatening to rupture and produce peritonitis.

Is hospitalization necessary for all cases of salpingitis?

No. In the early stages of the disease, treatment can be carried out at home with safety. However, if response is inadequate, hospitalization is indicated.

Does salpingitis ever clear up by itself?

No. All cases must be treated intensively.

What are the chances of recovery from salpingitis?

Very few women die of salpingitis, but the chronic form of the disease can be cured only by removal of the tubes. In the acute stage, salpingitis can be cured if treatment is started quickly and is pursued vigorously.

Can the antibiotics cure a chronic or persistent abscess within the Fallopian tubes?

Usually not. Once a chronic abscess has formed, the only satisfactory method of treatment is the removal of the tube.

What kind of surgery is performed for salpingitis?

In disease restricted to one tube, simple removal of that tube is carried out. In more advanced disease, it may be necessary to remove both tubes, the tubes and the ovaries, or both tubes along with the ovaries and the uterus.

Is operation for the removal of an inflamed tube a major operative procedure?

Yes. It is performed through an incision in the lower abdomen, under general or spinal anesthesia.

How long a hospital stay is necessary after an operation upon the tube?

Approximately eight to ten days.

How soon after an operation upon the tubes can a patient get out of bed?

The day following surgery.

How long does it take these wounds to heal?

Approximately ten to twelve days.

Does recurrence of salpingitis ever take place after surgery?

Where radical surgery has been performed with the removal of the tubes, a recurrence will not take place. Where only one tube has been removed or where radical surgery has not been performed, it is possible for inflammation to return and involve the adjacent ovary or the other tube and ovary.

Is there a tendency for salpingitis to recur when it is treated medically?

Yes.

How often is salpingitis limited to one tube?

This situation occurs infrequently. In the majority of cases, the inflammation affects both tubes. However, removal of both tubes is not always necessary, as it is sometimes possible to salvage one tube.

Will removal of the Fallopian tubes interfere with normal marital relations?

No.

Does removal of the Fallopian tubes cause change of life (menopause)?

No. It is only when the ovaries are removed along with the tubes that menopause follows.

How soon after an operation for the removal of one or both tubes can a patient do the following:

Bathe	Four weeks.
Perform household duties	One week.
Drive an automobile	Six weeks.
Resume marital relations	Six weeks.
Douche	Six weeks.
Return to work	Six weeks.

What is an ectopic (tubal) pregnancy?

It is a condition in which a fertilized egg implants in the wall of the Fallopian tube and starts to grow.

What causes ectopic (tubal) pregnancy?

a. Previous inflammation of the tube is by far the most common cause of ectopic pregnancy. Approximately 25 per cent of all cases occur in women who have had previous salpingitis.

b. Infection following abortion, or infection following the delivery of a child.

c. Ovarian or uterine tumors which have produced mechanical compression, distortion, or blockage of a tube.

d. Previous peritonitis (inflammation of the abdominal cavity) which has created adhesions of a tube and has distorted its channel.

e. A birth deformity of the tube.

f. Unknown causes in women who are otherwise perfectly normal.

How often does an ectopic pregnancy occur?

In approximately one out of every three to four hundred pregnancies.

How soon after the egg is fertilized can an ectopic pregnancy occur?

Immediately after its fertilization.

491

How soon after an ectopic pregnancy has taken place can a diagnosis be made?

Usually within four to six weeks.

What are the symptoms of an ectopic pregnancy?

In the early stages of an unruptured ectopic pregnancy, the patient usually misses a menstrual period but does have slight vaginal staining. Some pain develops in the lower abdomen, particularly after intercourse. All of the signs seen during early pregnancy, including morning sickness, breast enlargement, etc., may be present.

When an ectopic pregnancy ruptures, the above symptoms may be followed by severe shock, fainting, marked pallor, abdominal pain, pain in the shoulder region, and pressure in the rectum.

What causes the symptoms when an ectopic pregnancy ruptures?

There is actual rupture of the tube accompanied by great loss of blood into the abdominal cavity.

What is meant by the term "tubal abortion"?

This is a situation in which the fertilized egg or young embryo is expelled from the end of the tube into the abdominal cavity. In many

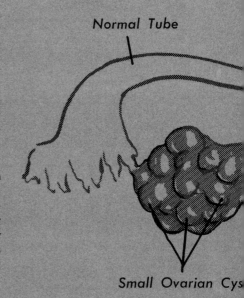

Ectopic Pregnancy / Cysts of Ovary. This is a composite diagram showing two distinctly separate conditions. On the left is pictured an ectopic or tubal pregnancy. An ectopic pregnancy usually only lasts a few weeks, terminating in rupture of the tube and severe hemorrhage which will require immediate emergency surgery. When ectopic pregnancy is diagnosed before rupture, the surgeon will operate and remove the involved fallopian tube.

The right side of this diagram shows an ovary involved in cyst formation. When ovarian cysts become larger than the size of a lemon or an orange and persist for any length of time, they are best treated by surgical removal. If the opposite ovary is normal, completely normal menstrual and reproductive functions will be maintained.

Normal Tube

Small Ovarian Cyst

of these cases the symptoms are not as severe as in a ruptured ectopic pregnancy, for the tube itself does not rupture and there is much less blood loss and shock.

Is the pregnancy test (A-Z test) always positive in ectopic pregnancy?

No. There are many cases in which the pregnancy test will be negative. This will depend upon whether the pregnancy is still viable (alive).

How does the gynecologist make the diagnosis of ectopic pregnancy?

By noting the appearance of the symptoms described above, associated with the presence of a pelvic mass in the region of the Fallopian tube. A positive pregnancy test will also help to establish a diagnosis.

In suspected cases, a needle may be inserted into the pelvic cavity through the vagina to note the presence of blood within the pelvic cavity. Or an instrument can be inserted from the vagina into the pelvic cavity to visualize the tubes.

What is the best method of treatment when an ectopic pregnancy is suspected?

If the diagnosis cannot be determined positively, the safest proce-

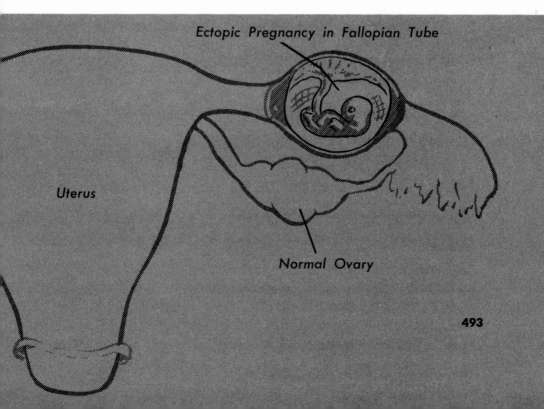

Ectopic Pregnancy in Fallopian Tube

Uterus

Normal Ovary

dure is to operate and examine the tubes under direct vision. Although this involves an abdominal operation, it is much safer to follow this procedure than to permit a patient to progress to a stage where the tube will rupture.

Is there any known method of preventing ectopic pregnancy?

No, except to treat all disease within the pelvis prior to permitting the patient to become pregnant.

What is the treatment for ectopic pregnancy?

a. When a definite diagnosis has been made, the patient should be operated upon immediately and the tube removed.
b. Blood transfusions should be given rapidly if there has been marked blood loss.
c. Suspected cases should be watched carefully and advised to call the physician should there be any change in their condition.

Are the ovaries removed when operating for ectopic pregnancy?

No, unless they are found to be diseased.

What is the greatest danger in ectopic pregnancy?

Hemorrhage!

What are the chances of recovery following ectopic pregnancy?

When modern facilities are available and prompt surgery is performed, practically all cases recover. A mortality of 4 per cent exists throughout the country, but this is due largely to the fact that many cases do not receive early surgery.

Is the operation itself a serious operation?

No more serious than the removal of a tube for any other reason.

What anesthesia is used?

General anesthesia.

How long a hospital stay is necessary after an ectopic pregnancy?

Eight to nine days. ·

What treatments are given prior to operating upon a patient with a ruptured ectopic?

Transfusions are given to get the patient out of shock and thus permit surgery.

Are there any special postoperative treatments necessary after an ectopic pregnancy?

No.

Is it possible for someone to have a normal pregnancy after an ectopic pregnancy?

Yes. The removal of one tube or ovary does not prevent a subsequent pregnancy, nor does it necessarily mean that another ectopic pregnancy will occur.

Are people who have had one ectopic pregnancy more prone to develop a second ectopic pregnancy?

To a certain degree, yes.

How soon after operation for an ectopic pregnancy can one become pregnant again?

It is wise to wait at least six months.

How soon after an ectopic pregnancy will menstrual periods return?

Usually in six to eight weeks.

Does cancer ever take place within the Fallopian tubes?

Yes, but it is an extremely rare condition.

What is the treatment for cancer of a Fallopian tube?

It is treated like any other pelvic cancer, by complete removal of the uterus, tubes, and ovaries.

Can cure take place after cancer of a tube?

Yes, provided that the disease has been eradicated before it has spread to other organs.

THE OVARIES

What are the ovaries?

They are a pair of almond-shaped glandular structures about one and one-half inches by one inch in diameter. They are located in the pelvis on either side of the uterus and are suspended from the posterior wall of the pelvis in close proximity to the funnel-shaped openings of the Fallopian tubes. Each ovary consists of an outer capsule which is grayish-white in color, a cortex or main substance, and a hilum or stalk through which the blood vessels enter and leave.

What are the functions of the ovaries?

a. The periodic production and discharge of a mature egg. The cortex of each ovary contains several thousand immature eggs, one of which matures and is discharged into the funnel-shaped opening of a Fallopian tube each month. *This process is called ovulation.* If the egg is fertilized by the male sperm, the process halts. If fertilization does not take place, menstruation follows. The interval between ovulation and menstruation is approximately fourteen days.

b. The ovaries manufacture and secrete sex hormones into the bloodstream. These hormones are called estrogen and progesterone. They regulate ovulation and menstruation, help to maintain pregnancy when it exists, and are responsible for the development of female characteristics. Thus, they are responsible for breast development, the female distribution of hair, the female figure, and the feminine voice.

Are both ovaries necessary for normal ovarian function?

No. Only one ovary, or part of an ovary, is necessary to maintain normal function.

At what age does the ovary begin to function?

From the onset of puberty at approximately twelve to fourteen years of age.

Is the ovary ever the site of inflammation or infection?

Yes. Because of its close proximity to the Fallopian tube, disease of that structure will frequently spread to the ovary.

What are the symptoms of an inflamed or infected ovary?

They are the same as those involving disease of the Fallopian tube (salpingitis).

What is meant by the term "ovarian dysfunction"?

It is a state in which there is disturbed ovarian hormone production or imbalance, characterized by upset in the menstrual cycle and in the ability to become pregnant or maintain pregnancy. Such disorders may originate within the ovary or they may be secondary to disturbed function within other endocrine glands, such as the pituitary or thyroid.

What are some of the symptoms which may develop with prolonged dysfunction of the ovaries?

a. Complete upset in the menstrual cycle and in the character and nature of menstruation.
b. Obesity.
c. The development of extra hair upon the body (hirsutism).
d. Overgrowth of the lining membrane of the uterus (endometrial hyperplasia).
e. Infertility (inability to become pregnant).

What are the results of ovarian dysfunction?

The normal balance between the production and utilization of its two main hormones, estrogen and progesterone, is disturbed. This may interfere with ovulation, menstruation, or with preparation of the uterus for the acceptance of a pregnancy.

What is the treatment for ovarian dysfunction?

First, the exact cause of the imbalance must be determined. Hormone studies of the blood and urine are carried out in an attempt to find the seat of the difficulty and to determine whether it originates in the

497

ovary, the thyroid, or the pituitary gland. Endometrial biopsy and vaginal smears are also performed as an aid to a precise diagnosis.

a. When cysts accompany ovarian dysfunction, an operation with removal of a wedge-shaped section from each ovary often helps to correct the disturbance.

b. X-ray radiation, in small doses to stimulate the ovaries to secrete, has been found to be helpful in certain cases.

c. When thyroid or pituitary gland dysfunction is found to be the cause of the ovarian disorder, the condition must be remedied by appropriate medication before the ovarian dysfunction can be corrected.

d. Cyclic therapy, the giving of regulated doses of estrogen and progesterone hormones, in a manner simulating the normal cycle, may prove beneficial.

e. More recently, cortisone has been found successful in certain cases in restoring normal ovarian function.

Does disturbed ovarian function ever subside by itself?

Yes. This occurs frequently without any treatment whatever.

Can pregnancy follow ovarian dysfunction?

If ovarian dysfunction is accompanied by lack of ovulation, the chances for pregnancy are nil. However, once the dysfunction is corrected, pregnancy may take place!

At what age may ovarian dysfunction occur?

It can take place at any age from puberty to menopause but is seen most often during the first years of adolescence or early adulthood.

What are follicle cysts?

These are small fluid-filled sacs appearing on the surface of an ovary. They arise from the failure of the egg-producing follicle to rupture. Thus, the cyst persists instead of being absorbed.

To what size do follicle cysts grow?

They may vary from the size of a pea to that of a plum.

What are the causes of follicle cysts?

   a. Previous infection which has produced a thickening of the outer coat of the ovary.

   b. Disturbance in ovarian function.

What symptoms do follicle cysts cause?

They may cause no symptoms, or they may result in ovarian dysfunction as described above. The larger solitary follicle cysts sometimes cause lower abdominal pain, urinary distress, pain on intercourse, and menstrual irregularity.

Do follicle cysts ever rupture?

Yes. When this happens, it may be accompanied by severe pain in the lower abdomen, tenderness on pressure, nausea, vomiting, or even a state of shock. It is often difficult for the gynecologist to distinguish a ruptured follicle cyst from appendicitis or from an ectopic pregnancy.

What is the treatment for follicle cysts?

Treatment is seldom required for the simple, small or multiple cysts which are associated with no symptoms. Multiple cysts which cause symptoms and are associated with ovarian dysfunction should be treated by surgery with the removal of wedge-shaped sections of the ovaries. If rupture or twist of a solitary cyst takes place, and the symptoms do not abate within a day or two, surgery may be necessary.

Do follicle cysts of the ovaries ever disappear by themselves?

Yes.

Is there a tendency for follicle cysts to recur?

Yes. Patients who have had follicle cysts require periodic observation by their gynecologists.

What is a corpus luteum cyst of the ovary?

After the egg has broken out of the ovary, the follicle is supposed to undergo shrinkage and disappear. In some cases, instead of disappearing, the follicle develops into a cyst (sac). Such a cyst may be

499

filled with blood and may enlarge to the size of a lemon, orange, or even larger.

What are the symptoms of a corpus luteum cyst?

It may cause no symptoms, or if it is large, it may cause pain, delay in menstruation, or painful intercourse. If the cyst ruptures, there may be acute onset of pain, nausea, vomiting, urinary disturbance, and severe pain in the lower abdomen. This may give the appearance of an acute surgical condition such as appendicitis or ectopic pregnancy and may demand surgery.

When is it necessary to operate upon a ruptured corpus luteum cyst?

If the symptoms persist or if there has been a great deal of blood loss.

Are there other types of ovarian cysts?

Yes. There are many types, including simple solitary cysts and cystic tumors.

Do these cysts ever grow to large size?

Yes. Some of them may fill the entire abdominal cavity and reach the size of a watermelon.

What is the treatment for these cysts?

Surgical removal as promptly as possible.

Are tumors of the ovary very common?

Yes.

What types of tumors affect the ovary?

a. Benign solid or cystic tumors.
b. Malignant solid or cystic tumors.
c. Hormone-producing tumors.

Why is the ovary so often the seat of tumor or cyst formation?

The eggs within the ovaries contain all the basic primitive cells which go into the formation of a new human being, and it is not surprising that some of these may undergo abnormal growth. Also, the ovary itself is subject to so many wide and varied fluctuations in function that it is not difficult to appreciate that things might go wrong and lead to tumor growth.

Do tumors of the ovary occur in women at any age?

Yes. They occur from earliest childhood to the latest years of life.

What is a dermoid cyst of the ovary?

This is a tumor occurring in women usually between the ages of twenty and fifty. It is frequently found in both ovaries and may grow to be as large as an orange. It is composed of many types of cells and may even include hair, bone, and teeth. Dermoid cysts also have been found to contain other tissues which resemble organs in a primitive stage of development.

Are dermoid cysts malignant?

The great majority are not malignant, but some will become malignant if they are not removed.

How is the diagnosis of a dermoid cyst made?

By pelvic examination and by x-ray examination.

What is the treatment for dermoid cyst of the ovary?

In the childbearing age, resection of the dermoid cyst. Past the childbearing age, removal of the ovary or ovaries and uterus.

What are hormone-producing tumors of the ovaries?

These are tumors which manufacture either female or male sex hormones in great excess. Thus, a tumor of the ovary which produces a male-type hormone will cause the patient to assume male characteristics, such as growth of hair on the face and chest, deepening of the voice, and loss of feminine appearance.

Are hormone-producing tumors of the ovary very common?

No.

What is the treatment for hormone-producing tumors of the ovary?

Age plays an important role. Surgical removal of the diseased ovary

501

is indicated in some cases; in older women, the uterus should also be removed.

Will altered characteristics disappear after removal of a hormone-producing ovarian tumor?

Yes.

What are fibromas of the ovary?

These are solid tumors constituting about 5 per cent of all ovarian growths. They are commonly associated with fluid secretion in the abdominal cavity and, because of their similarity to certain malignant growths of the ovary, they must be very carefully analyzed after being removed.

Does endometriosis affect the ovary?

Yes. In about one out of eight cases of endometriosis, the condition is found in the ovary. It is almost always associated with endometriosis elsewhere.

Is cancer of the ovary a common condition?

Unfortunately, yes. Cancers will appear as either solid or cystic growths and they may arise from one or from both ovaries. Cancer of the ovary may also develop from benign tumors of the ovaries such as dermoid cysts.

Does secondary cancer ever affect the ovary?

Yes. This is quite common and occurs from the spread of a cancer of the stomach, breast, or uterus.

At what age does cancer most commonly affect the ovary?

The highest incidence occurs in the years between forty and fifty, although it is sometimes found in young girls and in elderly women.

How does one make the diagnosis of cancer of the ovary?

By pelvic examination. Fluid in the abdominal cavity is a frequent finding suggestive of an ovarian malignancy.

502

What is the treatment for malignant tumors of the ovary?

The present mode of treatment involves surgery, with total and complete removal of the uterus, both tubes, both ovaries, and the ligaments and tissues surrounding these structures. Surgery is followed by x-ray treatment or the application of other radioactive substances in the majority of cases.

What are the possibilities of cure of cancer of the ovary?

If the patient is operated upon early, before there has been spread to other structures or organs, the chances are fairly good. Surgical recovery takes place in almost all cases, as these operations are not excessively dangerous.

Is cancer of the ovary ever permanently cured?

Yes; approximately one out of four women can be cured permanently.

Will a cancer smear from the vagina help to establish a diagnosis of cancer of the ovary?

In rare instances, yes.

What is the best method to prevent cancer of the ovary?

Frequent, periodic pelvic examinations will reveal the presence of abnormality in the ovary and alert the patient to the need for possible surgery. If surgery is performed early for suspicious tumors, many patients can be saved before the tumor has become malignant or before it has spread to other structures.

What is the best treatment for any ovarian cyst or tumor?

If it persists or shows signs of growth, operation should be performed to evaluate the exact nature of the lesion. In this way, many ovarian tumors can be removed which might have become malignant at some future date. Also, early removal of a persistently cystic or enlarged ovary will prevent it from twisting or rupturing.

Is medical treatment ever preferred to surgical treatment in tumors of the ovaries?

No.

What are some of the exact criteria for advising surgery for ovarian conditions?

    a. Any ovarian mass more than two inches in diameter which persists on repeated examination, should be removed.

    b. Any rapid growth of an ovarian tumor should be operated upon.

    c. The presence of free fluid within the abdominal cavity, in the presence of an ovarian tumor, should indicate surgery.

    d. The appearance of weight loss, anemia, weakness, in the presence of an ovarian tumor, should warrant surgery.

    e. Where endometrial hyperplasia is found in the presence of an ovarian mass, surgery is indicated.

Is it possible to determine, while the patient is on the operating table, whether a tumor of the ovary is malignant?

Yes. A pathologist will take a frozen section of a tumor and examine it under the microscope while the patient is on the operating table. This will determine whether or not the tumor is malignant and will suggest to the surgeon how extensive his operative procedure should be.

Do ovarian tumors ever occur during pregnancy?

Yes. Cysts of the ovary occasionally occur during pregnancy.

Do cysts which occur during pregnancy harm the embryo?

No.

Do ovarian cysts or tumors ever create an acute abdominal condition?

Yes, there is a great tendency for cysts or tumors of the ovary to twist upon their stalks. This will cause all of the signs of an acute abdominal condition and will require immediate surgery.

Do cysts of the ovary ever rupture?

Occasionally this happens, and when it does, emergency operation is indicated.

Does the removal of the ovaries alter one's sexual desires?

Not in the slightest.

How soon after operations upon the ovaries can one do the following:

Bathe	Two weeks.
Drive an automobile	Four weeks.
Resume household duties	Six weeks.
Return to work	Six weeks.
Resume marital relations	Six weeks.
Douche	Six weeks.

Can a woman become pregnant after the removal of one ovary?

Yes. This does not reduce her chances for pregnancy at all.

Does removal of both ovaries always bring on change of life (menopause)?

Yes, unless the woman has already passed the menopause.

Does a patient with only one ovary menstruate regularly?

Yes.

THE MENOPAUSE
(Change of Life)

What is the menopause?

It is that period in a woman's life during which ovulation (the production of mature eggs) and menstruation come to an end. It is commonly called "the change of life." In other words, menopause represents the natural aging process.

When does menopause occur?

In most women, between the ages of forty-five and fifty, but it may occur as early as thirty-five and as late as fifty-five years of age.

What is meant by the term "artificial menopause"?

It is a state created by the surgical removal of the ovaries or by x-ray treatments to the ovaries which cause them to cease ovulating.

What produces menopause?

A decrease and eventual stoppage in the secretion of hormones by the ovaries.

What are the reactions to menopause?

These vary widely. They may be absent or minimal; they may be marked and disabling. The most important factor in menopause is a woman's psychological attitude toward it. Women who, for one reason or another, wish to suffer, may unconsciously have severe menopausal symptoms. It is not uncommon for a woman to mimic her mother's reaction to menopause. If women are properly oriented and informed as to the menopause, and if they are emotionally stable, they will probably react mildly.

What are the usual general symptoms of menopause?

a. Hot flashes.
b. Cold sweats.
c. Headaches.
d. A feeling of fatigue.
e. Nervousness and a feeling of emotional strain and tension.
f. Depression and a feeling of inadequacy.

What are early specific symptoms of menopause?

Irregularity of menstrual periods and a diminished flow.

How can one distinguish between irregular bleeding due to menopause and that which is due to a tumor or other disorder within the pelvic organs?

If there is any doubt as to the cause of the irregularity of the menstrual flow, the gynecologist will investigate it by doing vaginal smears or by taking a biopsy of the tissue from the uterus or cervix. Frequently, he will recommend a curettage in order to determine the exact nature of the condition.

What is the usual duration of menopause?

It may last anywhere from a few months to a few years.

506

What is the treatment of menopause?

   a. The most important step in the treatment of menopause is to re-assure the patient and to inform her fully as to the nature of the condition.

   b. If the symptoms are not severe, the best treatment is no treatment.

   c. Hormone replacement should be given only when symptoms are severe and then only under the guidance of a competent gynecologist.

   d. Tranquilizing drugs and sedatives have proven helpful in relieving symptoms in some instances.

Can relief from the symptoms of menopause be obtained by the giving of ovarian hormones?

Yes, but this relief is temporary and should be given only as a last resort.

What are the drawbacks of giving hormones to relieve the symptoms of menopause?

It may induce further menstrual bleeding. This, in turn, may arouse suspicion that the bleeding is caused by a tumor rather than by change of life. Furthermore, menopause is a natural, inevitable process and, at best, its onset can merely be delayed.

Are the tranquilizing drugs efficient in relieving the symptoms of menopause?

Early reports seem to indicate that they can be very helpful.

Do the symptoms of menopause always subside after the passage of time?

Yes, within a few months to a few years.

Is it natural for emotionally disturbed women to have more severe and longer menopause?

Yes.

Does the desire for sexual relations change with the menopause?

No. After cessation of menstruation, sexual desire continues as previously. In some women, sexual desire is increased because the fear of pregnancy has been abolished.

Should there be any change in a woman's personal feminine hygiene after menopause?

No.

Is it natural for the voice to deepen and for hair to grow on the face and body with menopause?

Absolutely not.

Can pregnancy occur after the menopause?

No. When ovulation and menstruation have ceased, pregnancy will not take place.

For how long a period after the onset of menopause can pregnancy take place?

It is possible for pregnancy to take place during the first six months to one year of the menopause.

Are there any structural changes in the appearance of the ovaries or uterus following menopause?

They tend to undergo slight shrinkage in size, but this change is not significant.

What is the significance of vaginal bleeding after the menopause has been well established?

Bleeding which occurs six months after the period has stopped should always be looked upon as possible evidence of a tumor within the cervix or uterus. This must be investigated thoroughly.

Are a woman's abilities to think clearly and to be mentally alert just as great after the menopause as they were before?

Definitely, yes.

Is it common for women to lose their youthful appearance after the menopause?

No, except that one must realize that the menopause occurs at an age when the youthful appearance tends to wane. The loss of female hormone secretions, however, has very little to do with the physical appearance of a woman.

Is there a tendency to inherit early menopause or late menopause?

Yes.

Does an early menopause indicate that the life span will be short?

Definitely not. The menopause is no indication whatever of a woman's ability to live a long life.

24 *First Aid*

CHAPTER

In Emergencies

BITES
Animal or Human Bites

What is the first-aid treatment for animal or human bites?

These injuries usually consist of puncture wounds, jagged lacerations, or bruises. They should be treated quickly and thoroughly in the following manner:

a. Scrub and cleanse the wound with water and any good soap for a period of five to ten minutes.

b. Apply a sterile bandage, or if this is not immediately obtainable, a clean handkerchief.

c. Any animal bite which has punctured the skin should be treated immediately by a physician so that he may give tetanus antitoxin and antibiotics, and recommend anti-rabies injections, if indicated.

Are human bites particularly dangerous?

Yes, because the germs in the human mouth frequently produce very severe infections, often much worse than those caused by animal bites.

Should antiseptic solutions, such as iodine, be used in the first-aid treatment of animal or human bites?

No. Strong antiseptics may damage the tissues further and should not be used.

Are bites always sutured (stitched) by the physician?

No. In some instances, for fear of infection, such wounds are left wide open to drain and are not sutured until several days later.

Insect Bites

Are bites dangerous from such insects as fleas, sandflies, mosquitoes, wasps, hornets, bees, or chiggers?

If someone is allergic to the sting of these insects, such bites can be serious injuries requiring immediate treatment.

What is the first-aid treatment for insect bites?

a. If a sting has been left in place, this should be gently plucked out. It is important not to break it in attempts at removal.

b. If a person is known to be allergic to a particular type of bite and is bitten on an extremity, it might be well to place a tourniquet above the bite on the extremity, so that the absorption of the poison will take place more slowly. It is important not to allow a tourniquet to remain in place for more than twenty minutes at a time. Release it for ten minutes and then reapply.

c. Medical advice should be obtained if a great degree of swelling takes place. The physician will give an anti-allergic medication or will take other measures to counteract the effect of the bite.

d. It is important not to scratch a bite, as this will cause secondary infection and will lead to greater absorption of the poison.

Is a bite from a black widow spider a serious injury?

Yes, particularly when it affects young children. Occasional fatalities have been reported. Bites from these spiders are characterized by severe abdominal pain and boardlike stiffness of the abdominal muscles.

How can one recognize a black widow spider?

It has a rounded jet-black body with a red marking on its belly in the shape of an hourglass. This is the female of the species and the one to be avoided. The black widow male does not bite.

What is the first-aid treatment for a black widow spider bite?

a. It should be treated just like a snake bite, by making a crossed incision over the bite and sucking out the poison.

b. A tourniquet should be applied above the bite just tight enough to cut off the return circulation. The pulse should still be obtainable.

c. Medical consultation should be sought quickly, as there are counteracting medications to the bite of a black widow spider.

d. Physical exertion should be avoided as much as possible.

What should be done for the bite of other spiders, poisonous centipedes, scorpions, or tarantulas?

These should be treated similarly to a black widow spider bite.

Are the stings of centipedes, scorpions, or tarantulas very serious?

Usually not. The only time a sting from these insects endangers life is when it happens to a young infant or when the bite is on the face or neck. However, stings from these insects may produce severe temporary symptoms and great discomfort.

Snake Bites

What is the first-aid treatment for a snake bite?

Since it is not always possible to tell whether the snake is poisonous, precautions should be taken in all cases of snake bite. The following procedures should be carried out:

a. A tourniquet should be placed just above the site of the bite. This should be only tight enough to stop venous flow and should not cut off the pulse. Anything, such as a handkerchief, tie, or belt, can be used as a tourniquet. The tourniquet must be released every twenty minutes for a ten-minute interval.

b. A crossed incision should be made over the site of the bite, and the bite should be sucked out.

c. The patient should be put at absolute rest and should undergo as little physical exertion as possible.

d. Have the patient transported to the nearest hospital and, if possible, ascertain the type of snake which caused the bite.

What are some of the poisonous snakes commonly found in the United States?

The coral snake, the rattlesnake, the copperhead, and the moccasin.

Is alcohol a good remedy for snake bite?

Absolutely, no.

Are the bites of poisonous snakes always fatal?

On the contrary, the majority of adults recover from snake bites. This is especially true if they can be admitted to a hospital promptly for the administration of the appropriate antivenin. The danger is greater in children, as the snake poison is apt to be more overwhelming.

Scorpion. This photograph shows the type of scorpion found in this country. Although the sting of a scorpion can be very painful, it does not cause death. Scorpions are found most commonly in the southern states, Mexico, and Central America.

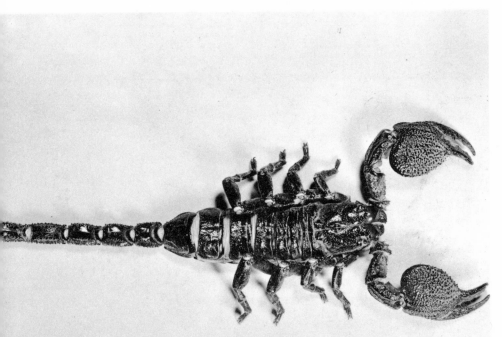

BURNS AND FROSTBITE

How are burns usually classified?

a. First-degree burns: These involve only the superficial layers of the skin and evidence themselves by mere reddening. Most sunburns are first degree.

b. Second-degree burns: These burns involve not only the superficial but the deeper layers of the skin. They are characterized by blisters and by the discharge of serum. Severe sunburns may fall into this category.

c. Third-degree burns: These burns involve all of the layers of the skin and usually have caused complete skin destruction.

d. Fourth-degree burns: This type not only destroys all layers of the skin but has involved the tissues beneath the skin, such as the subcutaneous tissues, muscles, tendons, blood vessels, bone, etc.

Second-Degree Burns. This photograph shows a second-degree burn of the arm. Such burns will usually heal within a period of a few days to a few weeks and will not require the application of skin grafts.

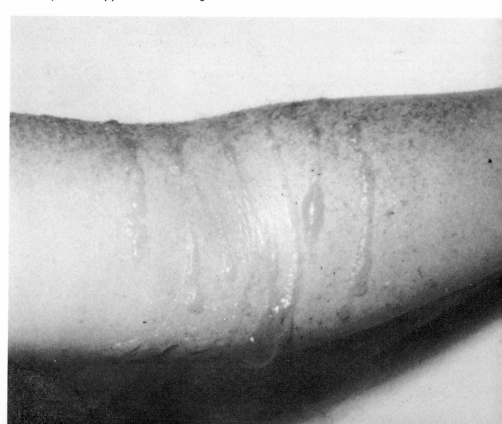

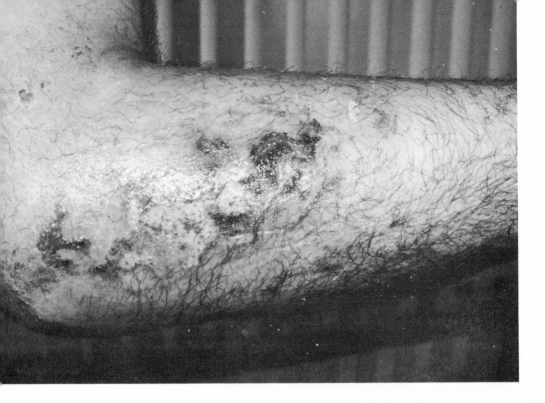

Burns. The photograph above shows an arm burn that has both second- and third-degree areas. A third-degree burn goes through all the layers of the skin, and if the area involved is extensive, it may require grafting.

Burns. Photo at right shows an arm with healed second- and third-degree burns. There are many different methods of treating burns, including the exposure method, which allows the burned areas to be open to the air, and the closed methods, which include the use of various ointments and bandages. The most important treatment for a burn is to see that the general health of the patient is maintained and that the burned area is kept clean. If a large area of the body is involved, the patient must be hospitalized and supportive measures such as the giving of blood, plasma, and antibiotics may have to be instituted.

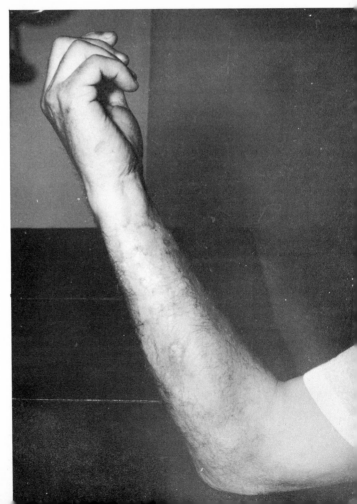

515

Are all burns caused by excessive heat?

No. There are many other types of burns, such as those caused by chemicals, alkalis, or strong acids. Also, some burns are caused by electricity or radiations such as x-ray, radioactive substances, etc.

What is the proper first-aid treatment for burns?

a. First-degree burns can be treated by any of the usual ointments which relieve pain and prevent the skin from drying or cracking. Most first-degree burns can be self-treated and do not require the advice of a physician unless the general health of the patient is also affected.

b. Second-degree burns must be treated by a physician. First-aid measures will include:

   1. Covering the area with a sterile dressing.
   2. Seeing that the patient maintains a large intake of fluids.
   3. Cleansing of the burned areas with large quantities of water and a mild soap.

c. Third-degree burns should never be self-treated. As a preliminary measure, dirt should be gently washed off with water, and a clean dressing applied. Large quantities of fluids should be given by mouth, and if the patient is in shock he should be immediately transported to a hospital on a stretcher. Ointments should *not* be applied to the burned area.

d. Fourth-degree burns should be treated in the same manner as third-degree burns.

Should the blisters of a second-degree burn be opened by the patient himself?

No. A physician should treat these blisters. Some physicians will open them while others will allow them to dry up by themselves.

Should people apply ointments to burns?

It is perhaps best not to apply an ointment to anything but a mild first-degree burn. There are various ways of treating a burn and many physicians do not believe in the application of ointments. Furthermore, the ointment which the patient prescribes for himself may not be the one the doctor may want used. It then becomes difficult to remove it in order to apply the proper medication.

516

Do chemical burns require special treatment?

Yes. It is wise to wash any chemically burned area thoroughly with large quantities of water in order to dilute the chemical and eliminate that which may still be in contact with the skin.

What should be done about the shock which accompanies burns?

Shock demands immediate treatment. (See section on Shock in this chapter.)

Is any special first-aid treatment indicated for burns of the eye?

Yes. These burns should be irrigated thoroughly with water to dilute the agent which has produced the burn. Medical care should then be sought immediately.

Should butter or homemade remedies or greases be used on burns as a first-aid treatment?

No.

Frostbite

What is frostbite?

It is a burn caused by exposure to excessive cold.

What is the first-aid treatment for frostbite?

a. Treat the general condition of the patient by warming him and by giving him warm foods to eat and warm liquids to drink.
b. The patient must be thawed out gradually and not suddenly placed from a very cold into a very warm atmosphere.
c. Give medications to relieve any pain which may exist. Aspirin or similar medications are usually adequate.
d. The affected part should be brought back to use slowly and should be exercised, but should in no event be vigorously massaged or rubbed.
e. The frostbitten part should be covered with a dry, clean dressing.

How warm should a frostbitten part be made?

Ordinary room temperature is as warm as necessary.

Should snow be rubbed into a frozen part?

No.

Should antiseptics be applied to frozen areas?

No. They may cause further burn.

Are any medications helpful in aiding a part to return to normal circulation?

Yes, but they must be administered by a physician.

Can one determine the extent of the damage resulting from frostbite soon after it has occurred?

No. It may take several days to discover the full extent of the damage.

CONVULSIONS AND "FITS"

What is the first-aid treatment for someone who has had a convulsion or "fit"?

a. See that the patient does not further injure himself by striking his head or other parts of his body against hard objects.
b. Allow the patient to lie down and give him plenty of freedom. Do not attempt to restrain him.
c. Open a tight collar at the neck to allow easier breathing.
d. Lift up the chin to improve the breathing airway.
e. If it can be done easily, place a folded handkerchief between the patient's teeth to prevent tongue biting. (Do not place your fingers between the patient's teeth, as you may be bitten).

Should cold water be thrown on people who are having convulsions or "fits"?

No. This is improper treatment.

Do most people recover from convulsions or "fits"?

Yes, particularly if the convulsions are epileptic in origin. Convulsions due to a brain hemorrhage or tumor may lead to death.

Should small children with convulsions be immersed in water?

No. It is much better to allow these children to remain comfortably in bed.

Should a parent pick up a child having a convulsion and run with him to a physician?

No. Recovery takes place in almost all cases of childhood convulsions. The best treatment is to allow the child to lie in bed unmolested.

Is there any way to find out how to aid a person having a convulsion?

Yes. In many instances people subject to convulsions will carry in their clothing instructions concerning their condition. Diabetics may carry instructions on what to do for them if they go into insulin shock. Epileptics often carry explicit instructions as to how they should be treated if they have a seizure.

What after-treatment is necessary for people who emerge from a convulsion or fit?

It usually takes quite a little time before they re-establish their normal thinking processes. Therefore, they should not be abandoned as soon as the convulsion has subsided. Many of these people will need quite a few minutes to know where they are and to realize what has happened. Stay with them until they regain their normal state completely.

DROWNING

What are the first-aid measures to be taken in cases of drowning?

After the patient has been removed from the water, he should be placed on his abdomen with his head turned to one side. Artificial respiration should then be administered by the first aider. He should kneel over the patient and compress his posterior lower chest rhythmically at the rate of ten to twenty times per minute. Medical attention should be obtained as soon as possible.

How long should artificial respiration be continued in cases of drowning?

As long as any heartbeat or pulse is obtainable. This is often for a period of several hours.

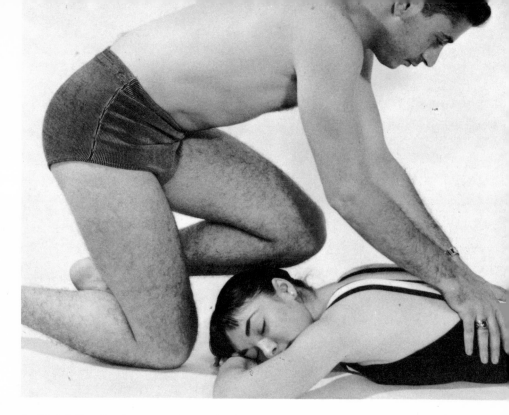

Artificial Respiration. In this method, pressure is being placed upon the lower chest, causing exhalation of air from the lungs.

Artificial Respiration. The photograph below shows the arms being raised and pulled, thus causing the chest cage to expand with resultant inhalation of air. Artificial respiration should be carried out rhythmically and slowly, with no more than 20 respirations per minute.

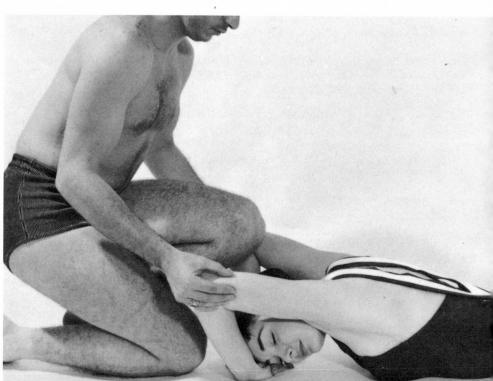

Is the mouth-to-mouth breathing method of artificial respiration beneficial in cases of drowning?

Yes, but it is easier for the victim to expel water from the lungs when he is in a prone position. After water has been expelled, mouth-to-mouth breathing can be started.

Is drowning always caused by too much water in the lungs?

Not always. Many cases of drowning are caused by spasm of the larynx and can be relieved by overcoming the spasm. There are many cases on record in which life has been saved by the performance of a tracheotomy below the point of the laryngeal spasm.

Should tracheotomy be performed by a first aider?

No, unless it is almost certain that medical attention cannot be obtained or that the patient will die before it arrives.

Does it help to turn a drowning person upside down and to hold him in this position?

Usually not. He will bring up water from his lungs if merely permitted to lie in a prone position.

When should artificial respiration be abandoned?

When the patient no longer has a heartbeat and is obviously dead.

ELECTRIC SHOCK

What is the first-aid treatment for electric shock?

Do not touch a person who is still in contact with an electric wire! This may cause your death as well as his. The patient should be removed from electric contact as quickly as possible. This may be accomplished by cutting off the current which is going to the patient or by disconnecting the patient from the wire contact by use of a dry stick or rope which is thrown around him. An axe may be available to cut the wire which is causing the contact with the patient. When using an axe, be sure that your hands are dry and that the wood handle of the axe is dry.

521

What treatment should be carried out for electric shock after the patient has been disconnected from electric contact?

a. Artificial respiration should be instituted as soon as possible.
b. The patient should be kept quiet and warm and supplied with oxygen if this is available.
c. The burned area which is often present at the site of contact must be treated in the same manner as any burn.

FAINTING, DIZZINESS, AND VERTIGO

What is the first-aid treatment for fainting, dizziness, or vertigo?

a. Place the patient in a lying-down position with his face up and his head at body level or slightly lower than the level of the rest of his body.
b. Raise the legs slightly above the level of the rest of the body.
c. If there is a tight collar or tie, loosen it so that the patient can get plenty of air.
d. If breathing is shallow, it can be improved by artificial respiration.

How long should a patient be kept in a supine position after he has fainted or after an attack of vertigo has taken place?

Until he is fully recovered and feels himself again. This may take anywhere from a few minutes to a half or three-quarters of an hour.

Is it common for people to faint a second time soon after they have recovered?

No, but they should be observed for a considerable time before being permitted to proceed on their own.

Do people ever die in a faint?

This almost never takes place unless a person has struck his head violently in the process of fainting and has sustained a fatal head injury.

Should cold water be thrown upon people who have fainted?

No.

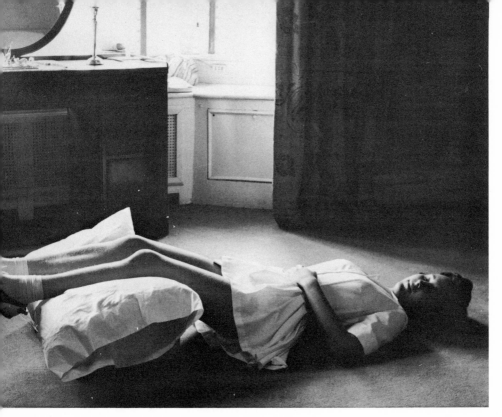

Fainting. This photograph shows the proper position in which to place someone who has fainted. By slightly elevating the legs, blood from the lower extremities can be made to gravitate back toward the head, where it is needed. Fainting is thought to be caused by constriction of the blood vessels which go to the brain. By keeping the head at the level of the rest of the body or slightly below it, blood will flow in larger quantities toward the brain and consciousness will be restored.

Do people who faint or who have attacks of dizziness or vertigo usually recover by themselves?

Yes, without any treatment other than being permitted to lie down for several minutes.

FOREIGN BODIES

What should be done in the way of first-aid treatment for foreign bodies?

a. *Eyes.* Only the most superficial foreign bodies should be removed from the eyes by non-physicians. If medical care is not readily available, the eye should be irrigated with lukewarm water, or

523

a moist piece of cotton can be used to brush out the foreign body. A little bit of mineral oil instilled into the eye will relieve most of the irritation. Avoid rubbing the eye and avoid trying to scrape out a foreign body with any hard object.

b. *Nose.* If one can get the patient to sneeze, the foreign body will often be extruded. This can be accomplished by having him inhale some pepper through his nostrils or by tickling the opposite nostril.

c. *Ears.* Foreign bodies in the ear should not be attacked by lay people, as damage may result to this delicate structure. The best first aid is to place some olive oil, mineral oil, or castor oil into the ear and let it stay there for a few minutes. This will usually bring out the foreign body. No great harm will result from a foreign body remaining in the ear until medical attention is obtained.

d. *Splinters.* Only those splinters which can be grasped firmly by a protruding end and can be gently withdrawn should be attacked by laymen. Soft splinters or broken-off splinters should be treated by physicians. If a piece of foreign body is allowed to remain in the skin it will usually become infected. If medical care is not available, warm soaks for a period of a few days will often bring a splinter to a position where it can be withdrawn with a pair of tweezers.

e. *Stab wounds* (knives, shrapnel, or other weapons): Protruding objects of this type should usually be left in place until medical care can be obtained. Removal by non-physicians may result in severe hemorrhage. The best first aid is to place a sterile dressing over the area and transport the patient to the nearest hospital.

What should be done about pieces of clothing or dirt which have gotten into an abrasion or laceration?

Thorough washing with soap and water will usually dislodge such foreign bodies. This should be done as soon as possible after the injury. The injured area should then be covered with a clean dressing and medical attention should be obtained.

524

FRACTURES, DISLOCATIONS, SPRAINS

What is the first-aid treatment for fractures?

a. Keep the patient quiet and do not move the injured part until the extent of the injury has been determined.

b. Immobilize or splint the damaged extremity before moving the patient.

c. Always move the patient to a hospital in a lying-down position. Never sit the patient up or bend or move the injured part any more than is absolutely necessary.

What should one do if a splint is not available?

There is always a piece of wood or a stick or some straight firm object which can be used as an improvised splint. Furthermore, a fractured arm can be splinted against the body and a fractured leg can be splinted against the other leg.

Should the splint be padded before being placed alongside a fractured extremity?

Yes. A piece of clothing placed between the injured extremity and the splint will prevent injury from undue pressure.

How should a splint be kept in place?

By tying handkerchiefs at various places along the splint or by tearing up a shirt and using it as a bandage.

Before applying a splint, what should be done with the fractured limb?

Try to place it in as straight a position as possible. Do it gently so as not to hurt the patient.

What are the best positions in which to splint an arm?

In a straight position; or the arm can be strapped to the side of the body. In this way, the body itself acts as a splint.

What is the best way to splint a leg?

The opposite leg can be used as a splint so that the injured leg can

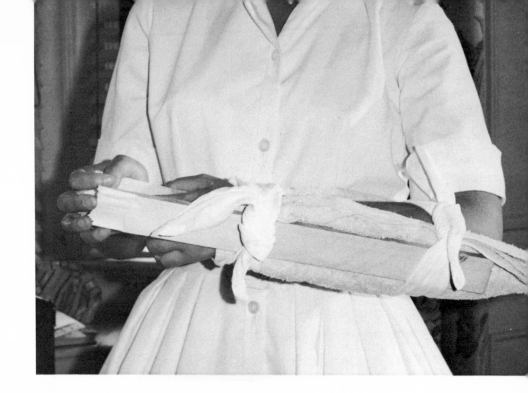

Fracture Splint. The photograph above shows a makeshift splint for a fractured arm. The only materials required are two pieces of wood, two ordinary towels, and two ordinary handkerchiefs. Such splints will prevent the fracture fragments from moving until definite care can be given by the orthopedist.

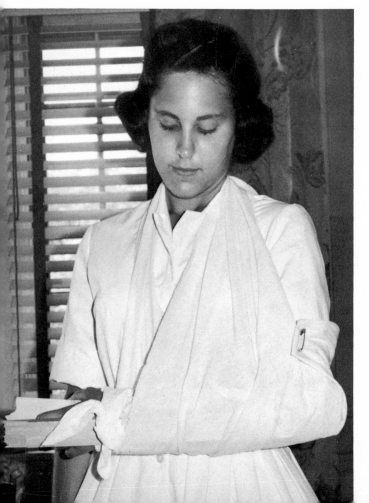

At left, a sling is being placed over an arm splint. It is usually best to transport the patient with his arm in a sling, so that the dead weight of the arm does not cause added pain.

526

be straightened and attached to the other leg. This will form an excellent splint in most instances.

Are special first-aid measures needed in the treatment of compound fractures?

a. Yes, the wound must be covered with a clean dressing or, if none is available, a clean handkerchief.

b. If there is severe hemorrhage from a compound fracture, it may be necessary to apply a tourniquet temporarily.

c. The limb should be splinted but no attempt should be made to alter the position of the broken fragments.

How long can a tourniquet be safely left in place?

A tourniquet must be released every twenty minutes, for a few minutes, to restore circulation.

Fracture Splint. Here is a makeshift leg splint made with two pieces of wood, two towels, three ordinary belts, and a handkerchief. A blanket or overcoat makes an excellent makeshift stretcher on which to carry a patient with a fractured leg.

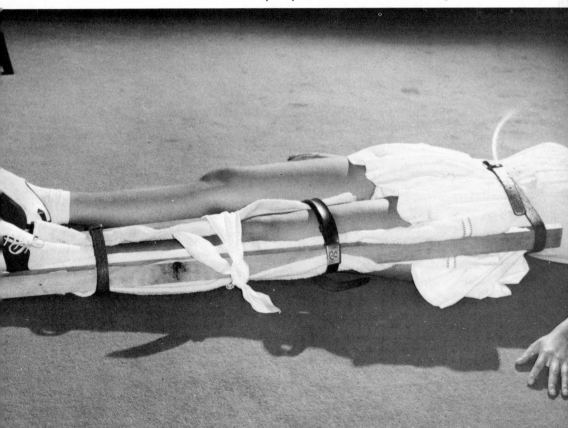

What special first-aid treatment is necessary for a fractured skull?

    a. The patient should be placed on his back with his head flat.

    b. The patient should be kept still and not allowed to move about.

    c. The patient should be kept warm and transported to the hospital as soon as possible.

Should whiskey or pain-killing drugs be given to a patient with a possible fractured skull?

No. This may do definite harm and should not be given.

Should fractures of the bones of the face be treated as potential fractured skulls?

Yes. A fractured bone in the face is often accompanied by a fractured skull.

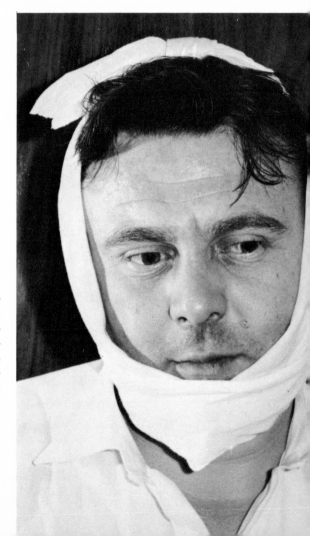

Fractured Jaw. This picture demonstrates how to apply a splint for a fractured jaw. Two handkerchiefs or towels or bandannas are the only materials required. The jaws should be kept together and the patient should do as little talking as possible, in order not to disturb the fracture fragments.

528

What is the best first-aid treatment for a fractured jaw?

a. Close the mouth so that the teeth come together as closely as possible.

b. Tie a handkerchief so that it circles the head from under the chin to the top of the head.

c. Allow the patient to remain in a sitting-up position.

What is the best first-aid treatment for a fractured shoulder or a fractured collarbone?

Place the hand on the chest in a comfortable position and tie a shirt or necktie around the entire body, keeping the arm and hand close to the chest wall. This will act as a splint and prevent motion in the fractured area.

Is it safe to immobilize a fractured limb in the position which is most comfortable for the patient?

Yes. This is safer than attempting forcibly to straighten out an extremity.

Should people with severe injuries to a lower extremity be permitted to walk or bear weight on the extremity?

No. When in doubt as to whether a fracture exists, do not permit weight-bearing.

How can one distinguish between a severe sprain and a fracture?

It is not always possible to make this distinction. It is wisest, therefore, to treat all severe injuries as if they are fractures.

What is the first-aid treatment for a dislocation?

Non-physicians should not try to correct dislocations but should immobilize the affected part and take the patient to a hospital as soon as possible.

Is it safe to pull or stretch a dislocated shoulder or finger?

This should be done only if medical attention is unavailable.

529

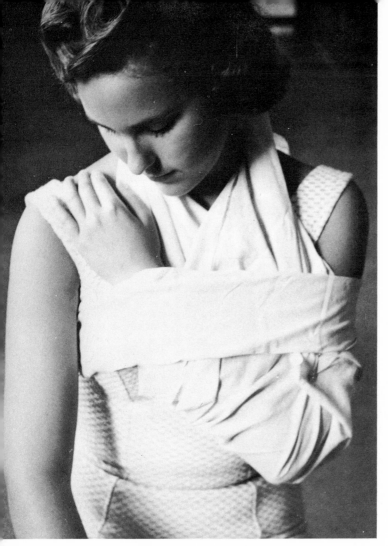

Shoulder Splint. This photograph shows the type of bandage used for a fractured shoulder or collarbone. Such a bandage will be effective for several hours, allowing time for the patient to be taken to a hospital or to an orthopedist.

Neck Fracture. Splinting a patient with a possible fractured neck, before taking him to a hospital. As little movement as possible is advocated for people who have a possible fracture of the neck or back, so as to avoid any unnecessary injury to the delicate nerves within the spinal cord. If there is doubt as to the extent of injury in this type of case, it is better to wait until experts arrive on the scene, rather than to move people in a manner that may produce further damage to the spinal cord.

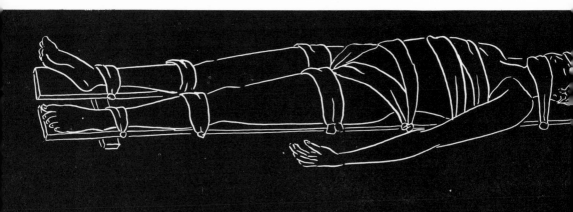

What special first-aid treatment is indicated for neck injuries?

If there is a severe neck injury, the patient should be transported, flat on his back, on a board, to the hospital. It is important to avoid twisting the body or bending the neck.

Is it necessary to keep the head rigid and not allow flexing of the neck if there is an injury in this area?

Yes. This is absolutely essential in order to prevent movements of the vertebrae. Movement may press upon the nerves in the spinal cord and cause paralysis.

What is the best way to avoid neck movement?

Someone should hold the head rigid by placing the palms of his hands firmly against the sides of the injured person's face and head.

What special first aid is required for a possible fracture of the back?

People with back injuries should be transported to a hospital lying flat, face downward. A board should be obtained, or a blanket can be used as a stretcher.

Is it safer to keep a patient at the scene of an accident until medical attention arrives, or should immediate transportation to a hospital be attempted in the case of a severe fracture?

If possible, wait for medical help before moving the patient, as serious damage can result from improper methods of transportation. Not all fractures are so urgent that the patient must be moved within a few minutes after their occurrence.

GAS POISONING

What is the first-aid treatment for gas poisoning?

a. Shut off the gas and open the windows.

b. Get the patient out into the open where he can breathe fresh air.

c. Mouth-to-mouth breathing should be applied.

d. Loosen any tight collars or tight clothing.

e. Call for an emergency squad so that pure oxygen can be administered.

For how long a period should artificial respiration be continued?

As long as there is the slightest evidence of a pulse or heartbeat.

Do people who recover from gas poisoning require careful observation?

Yes. There may be serious mental disturbance as a consequence of the effect of the gas poisoning upon the brain cells.

HEAT STROKE AND HEAT EXHAUSTION

What is heat stroke?

It is sunstroke, caused by overexposure to sun and extremely high temperatures.

Who is most likely to be affected by heat stroke?

Older people and those who are not in good health; men seem to be more readily affected than women.

What are the characteristic symptoms and results of heat stroke?

The patient runs an extremely high fever which may cause extensive damage to important structures such as the brain, the liver, or the kidneys.

What is the first-aid treatment for heat stroke?

a. Place the patient in a tub of cold water, preferably containing ice. This will reduce the body temperature.
b. Wrap the patient in cold, wet sheets or towels.
c. Give an enema containing iced water.
d. Summon the doctor as quickly as possible. People whose temperatures remain much above 106°F. for prolonged periods usually do not recover.

What is heat exhaustion?

This is a condition caused by excessive exposure to heat, not necessarily in the sun, in which the patient perspires, becomes weak, and may faint or lose consciousness. Heat exhaustion is more common in women than in men.

What is the first-aid treatment for heat exhaustion?

a. People suffering from heat exhaustion should be cooled quickly by being placed into a tub of cold water.

b. Salt tablets should be given. Ten grains three times a day is sufficient. (Heat exhaustion is always accompanied by free perspiration and loss of body salt.)

c. The patient should be kept in bed and allowed to rest until body fluids and salt have had time to be absorbed.

HEMORRHAGE

What is the best first-aid treatment for hemorrhage?

This will depend on the type of hemorrhage. If there is severe internal bleeding, such as may occur from an ulcer or tumor within the intestinal tract or hemorrhage secondary to the coughing up of large quantities of blood, the patient should be placed in a lying-down position and transported as quickly as possible to a hospital.

Are there any medications which should be given to a patient to stop bleeding from the intestinal tract or from the lungs?

This does not constitute first-aid treatment. Such people should receive expert medical care and it is perhaps best not to attempt to treat them before such care can be obtained.

What is the best treatment for external hemorrhage?

a. Place pressure directly on the wound! This can be accomplished by placing a sterile gauze dressing or a clean handkerchief on the bleeding points and pressing firmly with the flat of one's hand or with one's fingers.

b. If the bleeding is secondary to a very severe laceration in the arm

533

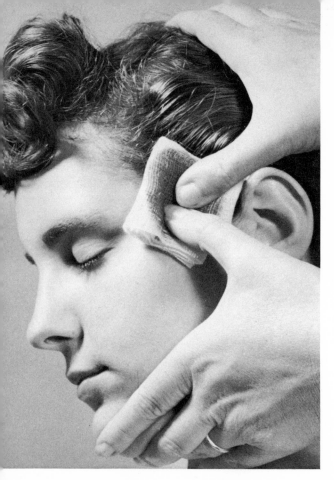

Direct Pressure for Bleeding. This photograph shows the application of direct pressure over a bleeding point in the forehead. Most bleeding can be checked temporarily by putting direct pressure over the spot which is bleeding. Note that a clean gauze bandage has been placed between the fingers and the bleeding point. If no bandage is available, a clean handkerchief may be used.

Direct Pressure for Bleeding Point in Neck. Life can often be saved by placing direct pressure upon a bleeding jugular vein. It is important, however, that the pressure be localized merely to the bleeding point and that pressure not be placed on the windpipe, which is in the midportion of the neck.

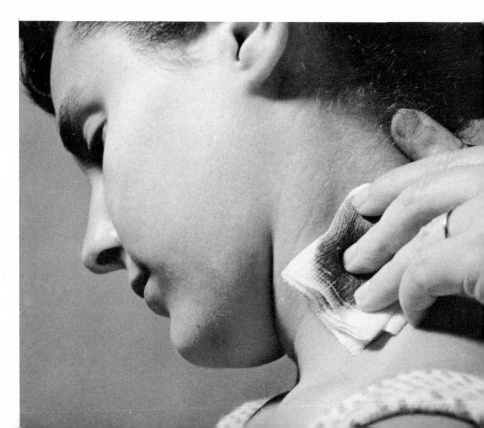

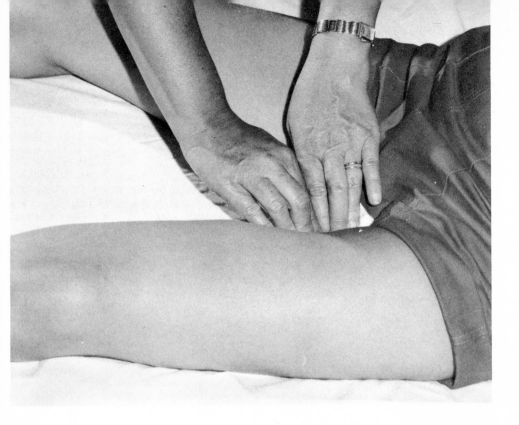

Above: Application of direct pressure over a bleeding point in the upper thigh.

Below: Direct pressure is being applied to a bleeding point on the lower thigh.

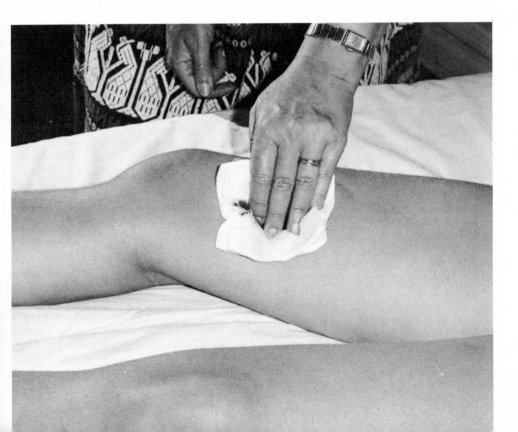

or in the leg, a tourniquet may be required. This is placed just above the site of the injury. It should be remembered that tourniquets must be removed every twenty minutes in order to allow the circulation to return.

How near to a wound should a tourniquet be applied?

As close as possible and just tight enough to stop the bleeding. If a tourniquet is applied too loosely, it will increase the amount of bleeding. If applied too tightly, it may unnecessarily damage tissues.

Does bleeding always start again after a tourniquet has been loosened for a few minutes?

No. It is often found that when a tourniquet has been in place twenty minutes, it can be removed permanently without resumption of hemorrhage.

Should a tight pressure dressing or tourniquet be applied in the region of the neck?

No. The best way to stop bleeding from the neck is to constrict the bleeding vessel with one's fingers.

Do people often bleed to death from external wounds?

No. Hemorrhages from the scalp, the face, or from one of the extremities usually look much worse than they are. It is rare for someone to bleed to death from the ordinary scalp or extremity wound, and most of these lacerations will stop bleeding by themselves within a few minutes.

In what position should people who have hemorrhaged be transported?

Usually lying flat or with the feet elevated. This will tend to combat shock by causing blood to gravitate toward the head.

Should alcohol or coffee be given to people who have had a severe hemorrhage?

It is perhaps best not to give any stimulants to those who have hemorrhaged. All efforts should be concentrated on getting the patient to the hospital.

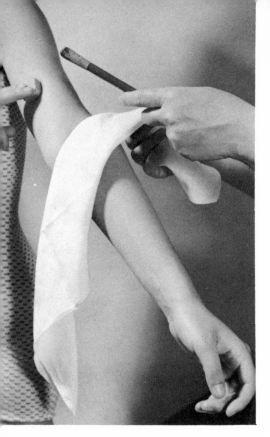

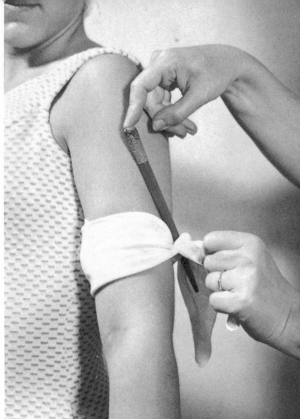

Tourniquet. This photograph, above left, demonstrates all the material required to make a tourniquet. A handkerchief, a penholder (or small stick), and an eraser are placed above a bleeding artery.

Above right: The handkerchief is tied loosely over the eraser and the penholder inserted into the knot.

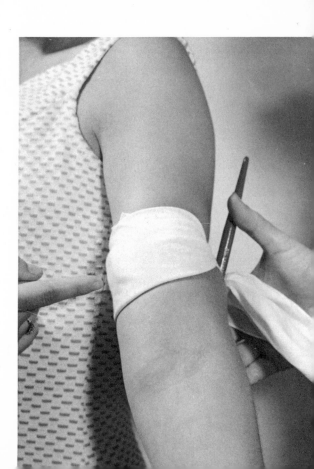

In the illustration at right, the tourniquet is tightened until the flow of blood is stopped. Tourniquets should be loosened every twenty minutes in order to permit blood flow to the rest of the extremity.

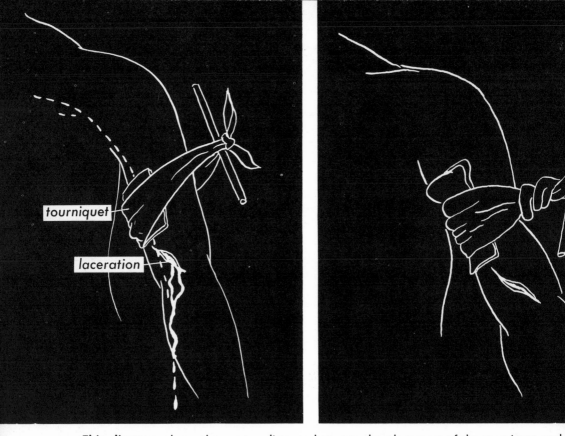

This diagram shows the proper distance between the placement of the tourniquet and the bleeding laceration.

LACERATIONS, ABRASIONS, AND CONTUSIONS

What is the first-aid treatment for lacerations, abrasions, and contusions?

a. Thorough cleansing of the wound with soap and water for five to ten minutes.

b. Direct pressure with a clean dressing in order to stop bleeding.

c. The application of a clean dressing and transportation of the patient to the nearest hospital or physician.

Should antiseptics such as alcohol, iodine, or mercurochrome be poured over abrasions, contusions, or lacerations?

No. It is found that these substances do more harm than good. The best insurance against infection is a thorough cleansing for a period of five to ten minutes with ordinary soap and tap water.

538

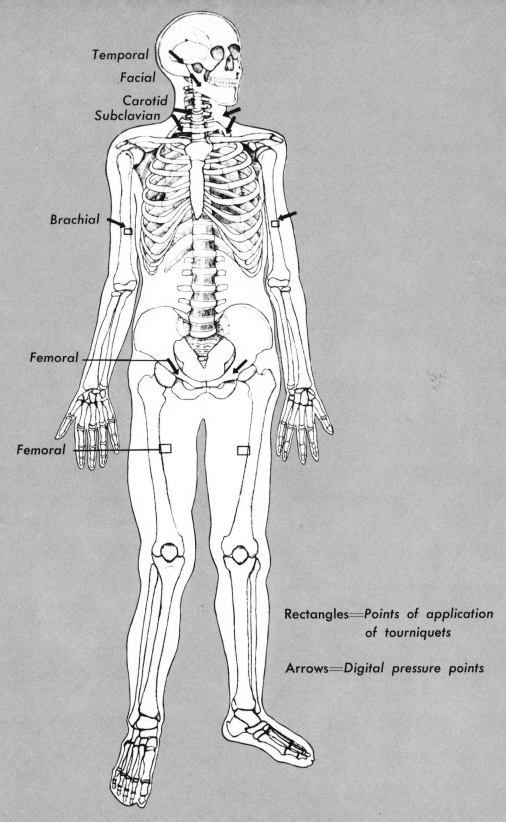

Temporal

Facial

Carotid

Subclavian

Brachial

Femoral

Femoral

Rectangles═Points of application
of tourniquets

Arrows═Digital pressure points

Pressure Points to Stop Bleeding from Major Arteries. These pressure points can
be located by noting the pulsations of the arteries at various spots throughout the body.

Will the application of ice to a bruise or contusion tend to lessen the amount of hemorrhage into the tissues?

Yes, but it should be remembered that damage can result if the ice is applied for too long a period of time. Ice should be applied for no longer than twenty minutes at one time and then discontinued for a similar period.

POISONS

What is the best first-aid treatment for swallowed poisons?

Empty the stomach as quickly as possible! This should be done by making the patient vomit.

What is the best means to bring about vomiting?

Have the patient drink several glasses of soapy water or a cup of water containing a teaspoonful of mustard or several glasses of salt water.

Is it wise to promote several episodes of vomiting?

Yes. As soon as the patient has vomited once, repeat the procedure in order to produce further vomiting.

What should be done after the patient has emptied his stomach thoroughly?

The best antidotes for almost all poisons are milk, the whites of several eggs, and strong tea. Give them in large quantities, and if the patient vomits again, give the milk, eggs, and tea again.

Is it ever harmful to give milk, white of egg, or tea as an antidote?

No. Although there may be more efficient and specific antidotes for some poisons, these substances cannot cause harm.

What other measures should be taken for people who have swallowed poisons?

a. If they are unconscious or are not breathing properly, artificial respiration should be given and they should be transported to a hospital.

b. The stomach contents should be saved for chemical analysis in order to discover the exact nature of the poison. This may determine what specific medications should be given as antidotes.

What poisons interfere with breathing?

One of the most common causes of depressed breathing is an overdose of barbiturates (sleeping pills). Artificial respiration should be given by the first aider in this type of case.

RADIATION EXPOSURE

What are the chances of being overexposed to nuclear radiation?

According to all experts, the danger of radiation poisoning is practically nil. Radioactive fall-out does not occur in inhabited areas in quantities sufficient to produce harmful effects.

What is the first-aid treatment when radiation exposure does take place?

If such an event should happen, the local authorities will give specific instructions to the population as to what first-aid measures should be carried out.

SHOCK

What are the symptoms of shock due to injury?

a. There may or may not be loss of consciousness.
b. The skin becomes a dull gray color and is cold and clammy to the touch.
c. The patient's body is covered with a fine perspiration.
d. The pulse is weak and rapid.
e. The pupils of the eyes are dilated.
f. Respirations are rapid and shallow.
g. The patient is apprehensive and complains of weakness and excessive thirst.

What is the first-aid treatment for shock?

   a. Place the patient on his back with his feet higher than his head.

   b. If there is any active bleeding which is contributing toward the shock, it should be stopped. (See section on Hemorrhage in this chapter.)

   c. The patient should be kept warm. Supply him with adequate blankets or other covering.

   d. If there is severe pain which can be relieved by the first aider, this should be done immediately. Pain is one of the strongest contributors toward the development of shock. If a fracture is present, this should be splinted.

   e. If it can be determined that there is no injury or wound to the abdomen, the patient may be given warm fluids to drink.

   f. The patient should be transported to a hospital as soon as possible.

Should alcohol be given as a stimulant to patients who are in shock?

No. This will only serve ultimately to increase the state of shock.

Should tea or coffee be given to people who are in shock?

No. In the time that it takes to obtain tea or coffee, the patient should really have had provisions made for transportation to a hospital where specific treatment can be instituted.

SUFFOCATION OR STRANGULATION

What is the best first-aid treatment for suffocation or strangulation?

   a. The patient should be placed in the open air.

   b. If there is anything about the neck that is obstructing breathing, it should be loosened immediately.

   c. Elevate the chin; this will give the patient a better airway.

   d. If strangulation is due to a foreign body which has lodged in the windpipe, the patient should be turned upside down and struck rather forcefully on the back of the chest.

   e. Encourage coughing to relieve the obstruction.

What is the best way to combat suffocation when a child has swallowed something "the wrong way"?

Place the index finger in his mouth and scrape around the back of the mouth. This will frequently result in the dislodging of the obstructing foreign body.

Should first aiders ever attempt to perform a tracheotomy?

Only under the most dire conditions, when it is obvious that the patient will die unless an opening is made into the neck. This should be done only when the patient can no longer breathe at all.

How does one perform an emergency tracheotomy?

By placing the fingers along the lower portion of the neck, the rings of the trachea can be felt. A sharp knife placed into the trachea will often relieve the strangulation and save a life. This, however, should never be done when medical attention can be obtained.

How long can people go without breathing and still maintain life?

No more than three to four minutes.

Should artificial respiration be carried out in suffocation?

Yes, provided the obstruction to the intake of air has been relieved. It will do no good to give artificial respiration if there is an obstruction to the intake of air into the lungs.

BANDAGING

What is the proper way to apply a bandage?

The photographs on the following pages illustrate the proper method of applying a bandage.

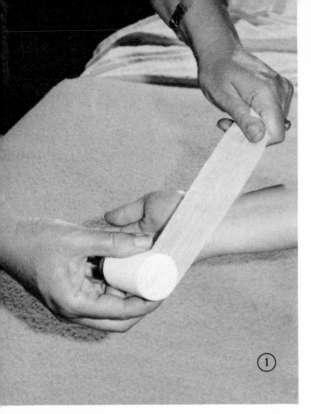

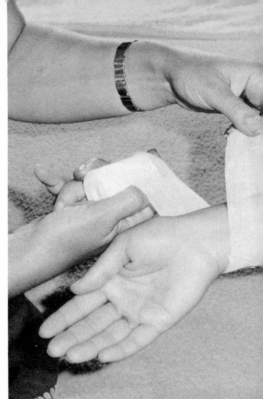

The Anchor: Starting the bandage.

The Anchor: The bandage is rolled around the wrist. Bandages should be applied snugly but never so tightly that they act as a tourniquet or cut off circulation.

The Anchor: The offset first turn is bent or twisted over the second turn.

The Anchor: A third turn locks the bent-over end firmly in place.

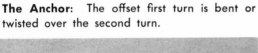

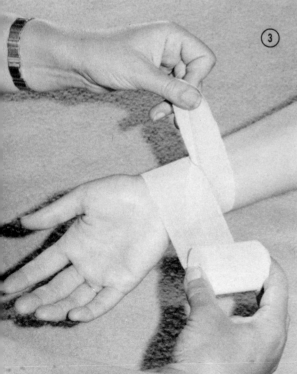

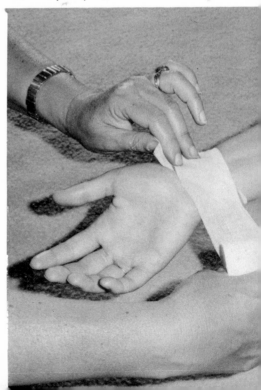

BANDAGING

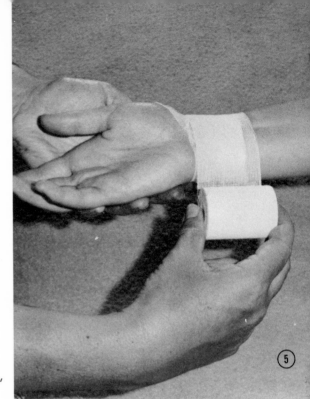

The Anchor is completed and the "roller" begun.

When the part of the body being bandaged is approximately uniform in size and shape, a simple roller bandage is used. Each turn should cover about two-thirds of the previous turn.

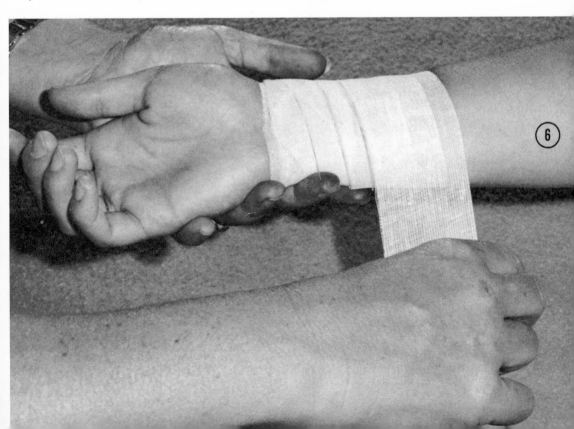

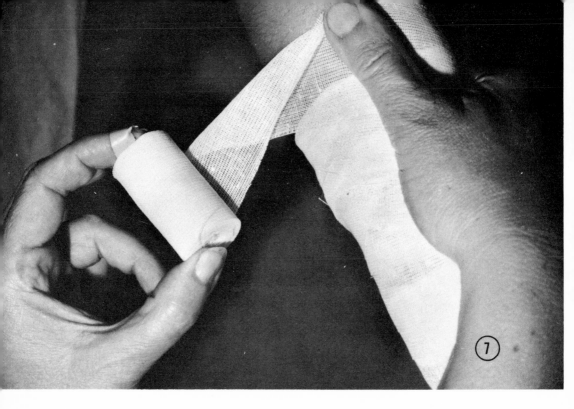

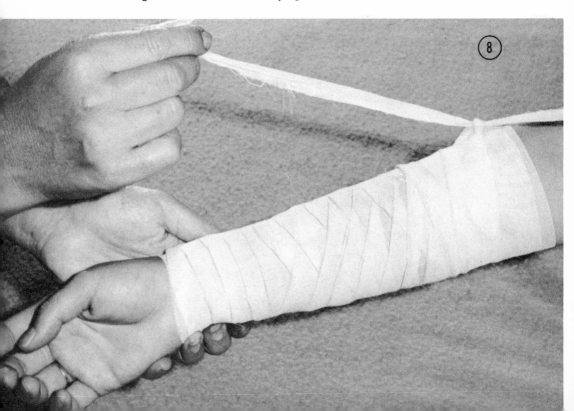

When the size or shape of the part is not uniform, the bandage is bent back on each turn so as to make it cling more tightly. This type of bandaging is called "the spiral reverse."

Bandages may be completed and fastened in place with adhesive tape or by splitting the bandage down the middle and tying it in a knot or bow.

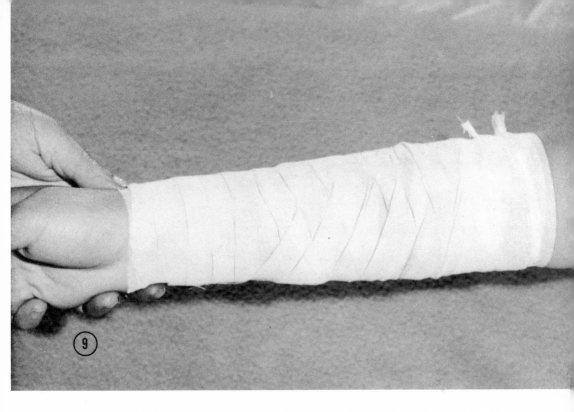

This photograph shows a completed bandage about to be tested for tightness.

No bandage should ever be considered finished until it has been determined that it is not too tight. This test can be carried out by placing a pen or pencil under the bandage next to the skin so as to make sure that circulation is not being impaired.

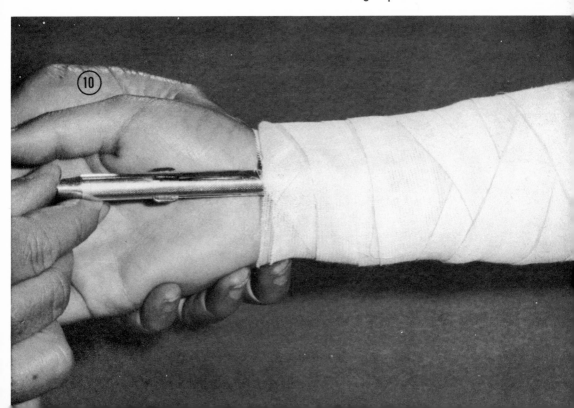

25

Gall Bladder
and Bile Ducts

Where is the gall bladder, and what is its function?

The gall bladder is a pear-shaped sac attached to the underside of the liver, beneath the ribs, in the right upper part of the abdomen. Its function is to receive bile, produced and secreted by the liver, and to store and concentrate it for use when needed in the processes of digestion.

For what types of food is bile particularly necessary in digestion?

Bile is essential for the digestion of fats, and fatlike substances.

How does bile reach the intestinal tract?

Through a system of ducts or tubes. The cystic duct leads from the gall bladder into the common bile duct. The common bile duct is the result of the joining of the two hepatic ducts which originate in the liver. Bile from the liver and the gall bladder travel down the common bile duct and enter into the intestine at the ampulla of Vater in the second portion of the duodenum.

If the liver produces and secretes bile, what is the special function of the gall bladder?

To store and concentrate bile so that an additional supply can be secreted into the intestine when it is needed after the eating of a meal.

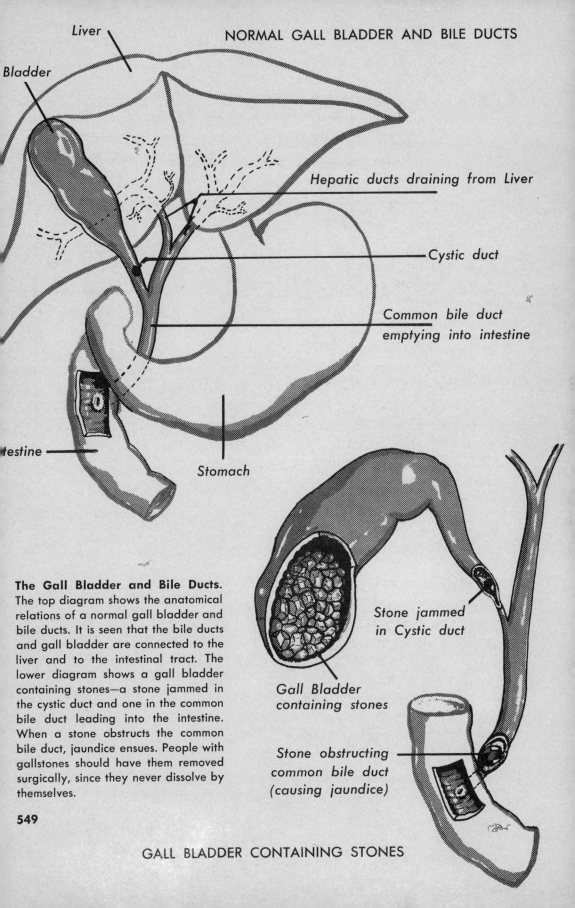

Liver

Bladder

Hepatic ducts draining from Liver

Cystic duct

Common bile duct
emptying into intestine

Intestine

Stomach

Stone jammed
in Cystic duct

Gall Bladder
containing stones

Stone obstructing
common bile duct
(causing jaundice)

The Gall Bladder and Bile Ducts.
The top diagram shows the anatomical
relations of a normal gall bladder and
bile ducts. It is seen that the bile ducts
and gall bladder are connected to the
liver and to the intestinal tract. The
lower diagram shows a gall bladder
containing stones—a stone jammed in
the cystic duct and one in the common
bile duct leading into the intestine.
When a stone obstructs the common
bile duct, jaundice ensues. People with
gallstones should have them removed
surgically, since they never dissolve by
themselves.

549

GALL BLADDER CONTAINING STONES

What foods often disagree with the individual who has a gall bladder disorder?

Any fried and greasy foods, French fried potatoes, heavy sauces, gravies, chicken or turkey skins, eggs fried in lard, turnips, cabbage, cauliflower, sprouts, radishes, certain raw fruits, etc.

Are disorders of the gall bladder and bile ducts very common?

It is generally agreed that disease of the gall bladder and malfunction of the sphincter at the end of the common duct constitute the most common cause of indigestion.

Is it necessary to operate upon the gall bladder very often?

Surgery for removal of a diseased gall bladder is the most frequently performed abdominal operation in people past middle life, and is one of the most common indications for surgery in all age groups.

What causes gall bladder disease?

a. Infection, with bacteria. This may result in an acute or chronic inflammation in the same manner that infection involves the appendix, tonsils, or any other organ.

b. A functional disturbance in which the gall bladder fails to empty when it is called upon to secrete bile.

c. A chemical disturbance causing stones to precipitate out from the bile. These stones may create an obstruction to the passage of bile along the ducts and into the intestinal tract.

Are gallstones always caused by an upset in chemistry within the gall bladder?

No. Gallstones may result from a chemical disturbance, or they may form as a result of infection within the gall bladder.

How prevalent are gallstones?

It is estimated that approximately one out of four women and one out of eight men will develop gallstones at some time or other before they reach sixty years of age.

Is there a special type of person who is most likely to develop gall bladder disease?

Yes. It is thought that the heavy-set type of person who eats a large amount of fats and greases is most likely to develop gall bladder disease. However, the condition is seen in all ages and in all types of people.

At what age does gall bladder disease first develop?

In the thirties and forties, although it is occasionally seen in younger people.

Does childbearing predispose one to the formation of gallstones?

Yes. Pregnancy produces a disturbance in fat and cholesterol metabolism. This is often followed by stone formation within a few months after the pregnancy has terminated.

Does gall bladder disease often take place *during* pregnancy?

Not very frequently. (It is seen most commonly in women who have had one or two children.)

Does gall bladder disease tend to run in families or to be inherited?

Only insofar as there is a tendency to inherit the type of body configuration, the type of chemical metabolism, and the type of eating habits that one's parents maintain.

What takes place when the gall bladder becomes acutely inflamed?

The blood supply to the wall of the gall bladder may be interfered with and the gall bladder may become filled with pus or its walls may undergo gangrenous changes as the result of inadequate circulation.

What causes most acute inflammation of the gall bladder?

A stone blocking the cystic duct.

What takes place when there is a chronic inflammation of the gall bladder?

Stones, resulting either from previous inflammation and infection or

551

from an upset in chemistry within the gall bladder, will be associated with a thickening and chronic inflammation of the gall bladder wall. This will lead to poor filling and emptying or even to non-functioning of the gall bladder.

What takes place when there is a functional disorder of the gall bladder or bile ducts?

This condition is characterized by failure of the gall bladder to empty and secrete bile when it is called upon to do so. Or there may be spasm at the outlet of the common bile duct which interferes with the free passage of bile into the intestinal tract. The patient has indigestion, heartburn, and an inability to digest fatty foods, greases, and certain raw fruits and vegetables.

Are functional disorders of the gall bladder usually accompanied by the formation of gallstones?

Not necessarily.

Is there any way to prevent gall bladder disease or the symptoms of a poorly functioning gall bladder?

Moderation in one's diet, with the eating of small quantities of fats, fried foods, and greases, will cut down on the demands made upon the gall bladder and may lessen the chances of symptoms due to inadequate function.

How can one tell if he has gall bladder disease?

a. Acute gall bladder disease (acute cholecystitis) is accompanied by an elevation in temperature, nausea, and vomiting, along with pain and tenderness in the right upper portion of the abdomen beneath the ribs. An x-ray of the gall bladder may reveal a non-functioning organ or may demonstrate the presence of stones. A blood count may show the presence of an acute inflammation.

b. Chronic gall bladder disease (chronic cholecystitis), when accompanied by stones, may cause excruciating attacks of colicky pain in the right upper portion of the abdomen. This is usually due to a stone being stuck in the cystic duct or bile duct. The pain often radiates to the right shoulder or through to the back.

There is nausea, vomiting, and tenderness in the abdomen, which may cease abruptly within a half-hour or so if the stone drops back into the gall bladder or passes through the obstructed duct. X-ray studies in chronic gall bladder disease usually show a non-functioning gall bladder and sometimes demonstrate the presence of gallstones.

c. Functional disturbances of the gall bladder evidence themselves by chronic indigestion; inability to digest fats, greases, and certain raw fruits and vegetables; and heartburn. X-ray studies in these cases may show poor filling and poor emptying of the gall bladder.

Is there a test which will make a positive diagnosis of gall bladder disease?

Yes, an x-ray test called a cholecystogram. This is done by giving the patient a specific dye in the form of pills. Some hours later, x-rays of the gall bladder are taken, and if the gall bladder is normal, the dye will fill up and outline the organ. The x-ray will also show emptying after the ingestion of a fatty meal. Sometimes, instead of giving the dye by mouth, it is injected into the veins prior to taking the x-rays.

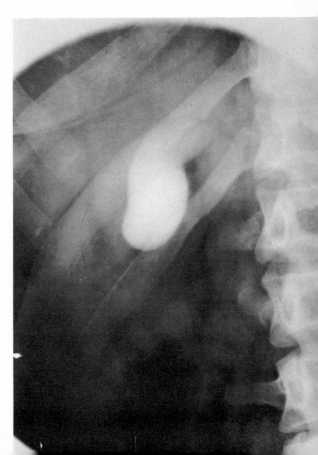

X-ray of a Normal Gall Bladder. In order to determine more accurately the presence of gall bladder disease, x-rays are taken after the giving of a medication which functions as a dye and, in the x-ray, lights up the interior of the gall bladder. If the gall bladder fails to light up or visualize, it indicates the presence of disease. Most stones appear as negative shadows in the x-rays.

What is the significance of a gall bladder not showing on gall bladder x-ray film?

This shows that the gall bladder is not functioning. Often, if the gall bladder fails to visualize with the dye, a second and larger dose of dye is given. Should the gall bladder not show with a double dose of dye, this is clear-cut evidence that the gall bladder is diseased.

Do gallstones always show on x-ray examination?

No. In some cases there may be many stones present and still they will not show on x-ray.

Can x-rays show stones in the bile ducts?

Yes. A relatively new diagnostic process called intravenous cholangiography will demonstrate stones in the bile ducts. This is performed by injecting the dye directly into a vein of the patient's arm and taking x-rays immediately thereafter.

Is this type of test dangerous?

No.

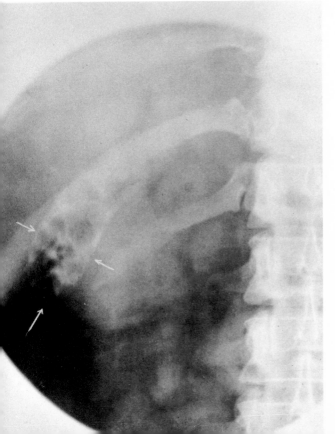

X-ray of a Gall Bladder Containing Stones. The stones in this x-ray show up as negative shadows surrounded by dye. Such a finding is a clear-cut indication for surgical removal of the gall bladder. This procedure (cholecystectomy) is safe and effective.

554

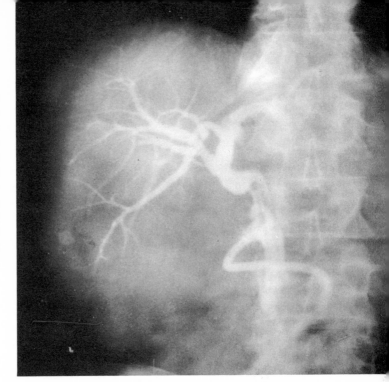

X-rays Showing the Outline of the Normal Bile Ducts Leading from the Liver into the Intestinal Tract. When the dye is injected into the veins, it travels to the bile ducts, and x-rays taken shortly thereafter show the lighting up of these structures. The outlines shown above would be distorted with negative shadows if gallstones were present.

How does a physician decide whether to advise medical or surgical treatment for gall bladder disease?

The functional disorders of the gall bladder, when not accompanied by stone formation, are best treated medically. All other disturbances of the gall bladder are best treated surgically.

Is the medical management for functional disorders of the gall bladder very helpful?

Yes, when the patient cooperates by adhering closely to a sensible diet and when the patient takes medications as needed.

Does a patient with gallstones always have to be operated upon?

Not in all instances. There are many people who have stones in their gall bladder that produce no symptoms. However, if gallstones cause any symptoms whatever, it is safer to operate than not to operate.

When is a gall bladder operation mandatory?

a. When the organ is acutely inflamed.
b. When the patient is suffering from repeated attacks of severe colicky pain due to the presence of stones.
c. When the gall bladder is known to have stones and the patient is

suffering from chronic indigestion, nausea, flatulence, and occasional pains in the abdomen.

d. When jaundice (yellow discoloration of the skin) occurs as a result of a stone obstructing the bile ducts.

What is the medical management for gall bladder disease?

a. The avoidance of those foods which produce indigestion, such as fats, greases, sauces, stuffings, and certain raw vegetables and raw fruits.

b. The eating of a bland well-rounded diet, with no large meals.

c. The use of certain medications to relieve spasm of the bile ducts and to reduce excess acidity in the stomach.

Does surgery always relieve the symptoms caused by a functional disorder when the gall bladder is known to be free of stones?

Although a certain percentage of these patients are benefited by gall bladder removal (cholecystectomy), others are not.

What can happen if an operation upon the gall bladder is not performed when indicated?

a. An acute inflammation of the gall bladder may progress to gangrene, with rupture of the organ. This may lead to peritonitis and possible death.

b. Recurring attacks of colic due to an obstructing gallstone may lead to the stone being passed into the common bile duct, where it will obstruct the passage of bile and cause jaundice.

c. If jaundice takes place because of an obstructing stone and surgery is not performed, the patient may die from liver damage and the toxic effects of prolonged bile obstruction.

Is jaundice always produced by gallstones?

No. There are many other causes for jaundice. The most common is hepatitis, an inflammation of the liver.

How can one tell whether jaundice is caused by an obstructing gallstone or some other cause?

There are many tests which help to make a conclusive diagnosis as to whether the jaundice is obstructive or is inflammatory in nature. A thorough history and physical examination, x-ray examinations, and several blood chemical tests will usually reveal the correct diagnosis.

Do stones predispose toward the formation of cancer in the gall bladder?

Yes. Approximately 2 per cent of those who have stones in the gall bladder will eventually develop a cancer. This is an important reason for advocating surgery upon gall bladders containing stones, regardless of the presence or absence of symptoms.

Is removal of the gall bladder (cholecystectomy) a dangerous operative procedure?

No. It is no more dangerous than the removal of an appendix.

Can gallstones be dissolved with medications?

No. Quacks and charlatans have claimed, for years, to be able to do this, but there is no satisfactory method by which stones may be dissolved.

When operating upon the gall bladder does the surgeon remove the entire organ or just the stones?

In almost all cases, the gall bladder is removed. However, there are occasional cases where the organ is so acutely inflamed and the patient so sick that the surgeon may decide merely to remove the stones and place a drain into the gall bladder. This procedure takes less time to perform and carries with it less risk.

Are the bile ducts removed when operating upon the gall bladder?

No. There must be a free passage of bile from the liver into the intestines. The bile ducts are therefore left in place.

How does the surgeon remove stones from the bile duct?

He makes a small incision into the duct, picks out the stone or stones with a specially designed instrument, and then drains the duct with a rubber tube (T-tube). This tube is removed anywhere from a few days to a few weeks later, depending upon the subsequent tests and x-ray findings.

557

How long does it take to perform a cholecystectomy (gall bladder removal)?

From three-quarters of an hour to one and one-half hours, depending upon the severity of the inflammatory process.

What type of anesthesia is used for gall bladder operations?

Either a general inhalation anesthesia or spinal anesthesia.

Is it common practice to remove the appendix while operating primarily for a gall bladder condition?

Yes, providing the gall bladder is not acutely inflamed. This practice is prophylactic and prevents a future attack of appendicitis.

What special preparations are necessary prior to gall bladder surgery?

Usually none for the patient being operated upon for a simple chronic inflammatory condition without jaundice. However, patients who have acute inflammation, or who are suffering from jaundice, require considerable special preoperative preparation.

What are the special preoperative measures used in these cases?

a. The passage of a tube through the nose to make sure that the stomach is empty at the time of surgery.
b. The giving of intravenous medications before operation in the form of fluids, glucose, certain vitamins, particularly vitamin K in the presence of jaundice to protect against possible postoperative hemorrhage.
c. The giving of antibiotics to the patient who has an acutely inflamed gall bladder or an inflammation of the bile ducts.

Are blood transfusions given in gall bladder operations?

Not usually; only in the most seriously sick and complicated cases.

Are private nurses necessary after gall bladder operations?

If the patient can afford it, a private nurse for two or three days will add greatly to his comfort.

How long a hospital stay is required?

Approximately nine days to two weeks.

Where are the incisions made for gall bladder disease?

Either a longitudinal incision in the right upper portion of the abdomen or an oblique incision beneath the rib cage on the right side is carried out for a distance of five to seven inches.

Are drains usually placed in gall bladder wounds?

Yes. One or two rubber drains will be inserted following surgery. These will stay in place anywhere from six to ten days.

Are gall bladder operations especially painful?

No. There may be some pain on deep breathing or coughing for a few days after surgery, but the operative wound is not exceptionally painful.

How soon after surgery can the patient get out of bed?

For the ordinary case, on the first or second postoperative day.

What special postoperative measures are carried out?

a. In the ordinary operation for a chronically inflamed gall bladder with stones, there are few special postoperative orders. The patient may eat the day after surgery, but fats, greases, raw fruits and vegetables should not be included. Antibiotics may be given if there is fear of infection. A stomach tube is sometimes passed through the nose and kept in place for the first day in order to avoid discomfort from distention.

b. The patient operated upon for an acute gall bladder inflammation or for jaundice will probably receive intravenous solutions, drainage of the stomach through a tube inserted through the nose, medications with vitamin K to counteract jaundice, and large doses of antibiotics for a few days. Occasionally, blood transfusions are also given.

How long does it take the average gall bladder wound to heal?

Anywhere from twelve to fourteen days.

Can a patient live in a normal way after removal of the gall bladder?

Yes.

What takes over the function of the gall bladder after it has been removed?

Bile continues to flow from the liver directly into the intestinal tract. The bile ducts take over many of the duties of the gall bladder.

Is it common for indigestion to persist for several weeks after removal of the gall bladder?

Yes.

Should a woman whose gall bladder has been removed allow herself to become pregnant again?

Yes, if she so desires.

Is it necessary to follow dietary precautions after gall bladder removal?

Yes. The patient should stay on the same kind of diet he followed before surgery, that is, a bland low-fat diet.

How soon after the removal of a stone from the common bile duct will jaundice disappear?

Within several weeks.

Do symptoms of gall bladder disease ever persist or recur after surgery?

Yes. Approximately 10 per cent of patients who have been operated upon for gall bladder disease will continue to have symptoms after surgery. These symptoms are thought to be caused by spasms of the lower end of the common bile duct (biliary dyskinesia).

Do patients ever form stones again after they have once been removed?

If the gall bladder has been removed they cannot re-form stones in the gall bladder. However, a very small percentage of patients may re-form stones in the common bile duct or in the stump of the cystic duct which has been left behind.

560

What treatment is carried out when patients re-form stones in the common bile duct?

Reoperation is necessary. This is a serious procedure but the great majority of people will recover.

Is there any way to prevent stones from re-forming?

Not really, except that one should guard against infection and follow a sane, sensible, bland low-fat diet.

Does gall bladder removal affect the life span?

Not at all.

What are the chances of recovery from a gall bladder operation?

The mortality rate from gall bladder surgery is less than 1 per cent. A fatality occurs mainly in the very complicated case, or in people who have neglected to seek treatment early.

How soon after a gall bladder operation can one do the following?

Bathe	In about two weeks.
Walk out in the street	Two weeks.
Walk up and down stairs	Two weeks.
Perform household duties	Five to six weeks.
Drive a car	Six weeks.
Resume marital relations	Four to five weeks.
Return to work	Five to six weeks.
Resume all physical activities	Six weeks.

How often should one return for a checkup after a gall bladder operation?

About six months after surgery and then again a year after surgery.

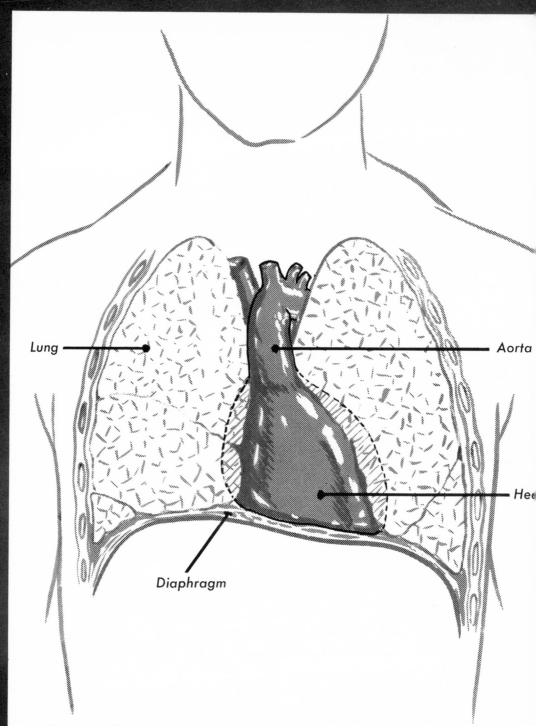

Lung

Aorta

He[art]

Diaphragm

The Normal Heart and Chest Cavity. Contrary to common belief, the heart tends to be more in the middle of the chest than on the left side, and as a matter of fact, part of it extends over toward the right chest cavity.

26 *The Heart*

What is the structure of the heart?

The heart is a hollow, globular, muscular organ composed of four compartments. It is divided into a left side and a right side, each of which has two connecting chambers—an atrium and a ventricle.

The right atrium receives blood supplied to it by two great veins —the inferior and superior vena cavas. These vessels carry to the right atrium the blood from all the veins of the body. This venous blood is dark-red in color, having a low proportion of oxygen, a high proportion of waste carbon dioxide and other products absorbed from the intestinal tract or manufactured by the tissues. From the right atrium, passing through a valve called the tricuspid valve, this blood travels to the right ventricle. From there, blood passes through another valve called the pulmonic valve, and then enters the blood vessels of the lungs. Here, the oxygen supply of the venous blood is replenished and the waste carbon dioxide is passed out into the exhaled air. From the lungs the reoxygenated blood passes on to the left side of the heart, first entering the left atrium. From there, it passes through another intervening valve called the mitral valve, and enters the powerful and muscular left ventricle. The left ventricle contracts forcefully and expels this fresh blood through the aortic valve into the largest artery of the body—the aorta. From there on, the reoxygenated blood is distributed to all the blood vessels and tissues of the body.

563

What is the function of the heart?

The heart is the motor, or main source of energy, which supplies the propelling force to keep the bloodstream in motion through all the blood vessels of the body. This organ, hardly larger than a fist, pumps an average of six thousand quarts of blood a day and can multiply its efforts manyfold when necessary. It beats incessantly during life, contracting at an average rate of seventy-eight times per minute, or approximately ten thousand times daily.

Poor heart action leads to poor circulation, which, in turn, leads to derangement and impairment of the function of the vital tissues of the body.

How can a doctor tell if a patient has a "good heart"?

He evaluates the heart on the basis of the patient's clinical history, the physical examination, and by other tests, such as fluoroscopy, x-ray, electrocardiography, which are carried out when additional investigation is indicated.

What is meant by the expression "a strong heart"?

Any heart which is normal in structure and which functions efficiently can be called "strong."

What is meant by the expression "a weak heart"?

A heart which functions inefficiently because of underlying disease or defect in structure.

Does heart trouble tend to be inherited or to run in families?

While certain conditions which attack the heart may tend to run in families, heart disease, by and large, is *not* inherited. The fact that one member of a family suffers from a heart ailment should not alarm related individuals about the condition of their own heart. However, it should serve as an additional incentive for these individuals to visit their physician regularly so that he may outline a preventive program, if indicated.

Does a patient with a "poor heart" ever develop a "strong heart"?

This depends upon the age of the individual as well as upon the

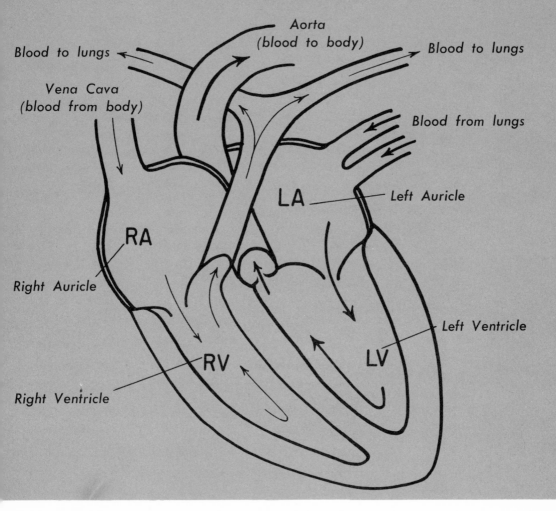

Blood to lungs

Aorta
(blood to body)

Blood to lungs

Vena Cava
(blood from body)

Blood from lungs

LA ——————— Left Auricle

RA

Right Auricle

Left Ventricle

RV

LV

Right Ventricle

Heart Chambers. This diagram illustrates the four chambers of the heart; the arrows indicate the direction of blood flow through the heart.

primary cause of the heart condition. Many types of heart trouble can be treated effectively, and in certain cases complete cure can result.

Do children with heart trouble ever outgrow it?

The term "outgrow" is one which physicians no longer use. The thought that a condition will clear up without treatment often encourages a negligent attitude rather than a positive approach to a heart problem. Strictly speaking, heart trouble is not outgrown. The popularity of this term had its origin in the fact that some heart murmurs heard in childhood were found to disappear later on in life. In actuality, these murmurs were not really indicative of true heart disease but were innocent atypical heart sounds. A true murmur indicative of an actual organic heart disease almost never disappears spontaneously.

Is strenuous physical exertion bad for someone with a normal heart?

Strenuous physical exertion probably has no significant harmful effect upon a normal heart.

Is strenuous physical exercise dangerous for someone with a "weak heart"?

Patients who suffer from heart disease should not indulge in strenuous physical exercise! This does not mean that such patients should make complete invalids of themselves. Rather, they should function within the range of limitations dictated by their own particular heart condition. The specific advice of their physician should be followed carefully.

What immediate effects does smoking tobacco have upon the heart?

In most instances, smoking will have no important harmful effect upon the normal heart. There are people, however, who show excessive sensitivity to tobacco. This may manifest itself by causing spasms of the coronary and other arteries, by creating irregularities in the rhythm of the heart, or by causing changes in the blood pressure.

People with heart diseases, especially coronary artery disease, should not smoke!

What long-range effects does smoking tobacco have upon the heart?

This issue is not yet decided. However, there have been interesting and provocative statistics recently to indicate that the incidence of coronary heart disease and other blood-vessel diseases is greater in smokers than in non-smokers.

Is drinking of alcohol bad for the heart?

Not particularly, unless drinking is excessive and prolonged.

Is it harmful to the heart to take aspirin?

No.

What medications in common usage are harmful to the heart?

Most of the commonly prescribed medications have no effect at all upon the heart.

Is excess emotional strain bad for the heart?

The normal heart will tolerate acute emotional as well as physical strain remarkably well. Whether *chronic* emotional strain will eventually cause heart disease is, at the present time, unanswerable. On the other hand, repeated or prolonged emotional strain is unquestionably deleterious to a heart whose function is already impaired by primary underlying disease.

Is there such a thing as a "broken heart"? In other words, can the heart be affected by grief or disappointment?

The term "broken heart" is, for all practical purposes, a purely poetic expression.

How can one tell if pain in the heart region is due to a heart condition or is due to trouble in some other organ?

Heart pain is an extremely variable symptom. It requires the skill of an experienced physician to evaluate whether a particular ache or pain actually arises from the heart. Frequently, he must resort to procedures such as electrocardiogram or x-ray to reinforce his clinical opinion.

Do people with normal hearts tend to outlive those who have heart trouble?

Other things being equal, yes.

How often should people have their heart examined?

People without a specific history of heart disease should not think in terms of having their heart checked. They should, rather, think in terms of a periodic comprehensive physical examination.

The patient with heart disease should have his heart examined at regular intervals, as advised by his physician. These intervals may vary greatly from patient to patient.

Do men have heart trouble more often than women?

Men have a much greater tendency toward diseases of the coronary arteries, and therefore are more prone to develop angina pectoris or coronary thrombosis. Other forms of heart disease are equally distributed between the sexes.

Do thin people tend to get heart conditions less frequently than stout people?

Statistically, the incidence of coronary artery disease is definitely greater among stout people. Other forms of heart disease do not appear to be appreciably greater among the stout. But it should be remembered that obesity puts an additional burden upon an already weakened or impaired heart.

Can doctors predict length of life by listening to the heart and making heart tests?

No. A doctor can merely determine whether a heart is functioning properly or whether it is diseased. However, in spite of all modern medical advances, it is impossible to make more than a rough guess as to the life span of the patient with a diseased heart. Certainly, there is no basis whatsoever for predictions of longevity in the patient with an apparently normal heart.

IMPAIRED HEART FUNCTION
AND HEART DISEASE

What are some of the common causes of impaired heart function and heart disease?

a. The heart muscle itself may be weakened so that it cannot contract with sufficient force. This may be caused by poor nourishment to the heart muscle tissue (as in disease of the arteries supplying the heart); or infection, inflammation, toxins, hormonal disorders or blood-mineral imbalance may weaken the muscle tissue of the heart.

b. The heart valves may not function properly—either because they do not open and close adequately or because they were defectively formed or absent as a result of a developmental birth deformity.

Heart valve disorders may be caused by acquired disease, the most common of which is rheumatic fever. Other less common causes of heart valve dysfunction are syphilis, bacterial infection, or diseases of the cell cementing substance.

c. Weakening of the heart muscle which has been overworked because of high blood pressure, chronic lung disease, endocrine gland disorders, anemia, abnormal connections between arteries and veins, or the above-mentioned valvular disorders.

d. Congenital (inborn) defects in the wall dividing the right and left side of the heart, as well as a great variety of bizarre inborn abnormalities of the heart and connecting great blood vessels. Fortunately, these birth deformities are quite rare.

e. Disease and abnormalities of the sheath of the heart, as in pericarditis.

f. Structural abnormalities of the chest cage and spine.

g. Disorders of the rhythmicity of the heart. Instead of beating regularly, the heart may adopt any of a variety of disorderly or abnormal rhythm patterns. As a result of these rhythm disorders, the heart is sometimes unable to pump blood efficiently.

h. Tumors of the heart may seriously interfere with good heart function. These tumors may arise in the heart tissue itself or they may spread to the heart from other organs. (Such tumors of the heart are a rare cause of cardiac impairment.)

What are the more common causes of heart disease?

a. Rheumatic fever.

b. High blood pressure.

c. Coronary artery disease (the coronary arteries are the blood vessels supplying blood to the heart muscle).

d. Chronic lung disease.

e. Congenital (inborn) heart abnormalities.

HEART FAILURE

What is heart failure?

Heart failure, medically known as "cardiac decompensation," may be caused by one or more of the conditions enumerated above. The term is applied when the heart is no longer able to accommodate to the normal circulatory requirements of the body.

Ordinarily, the human heart has sufficient reserve strength to compensate for most ordinary handicaps in the course of the above-mentioned disorders. However, as the disorder increases in severity and as the heart muscle becomes more and more fatigued, the heart becomes increasingly incapable of meeting its obligations.

What are the symptoms of heart failure?

a. Easy fatigability.

b. Shortness of breath, increased by mild exertion.

c. Swelling of the feet, ankles, and legs, usually increasing toward the end of the day and improving overnight.

d. Inability to lie flat in bed without becoming short of breath, thus requiring several cushions to prop up the head and chest.

e. Blueness of the lips, fingernails, and skin.

f. Accumulation of fluid in the abdomen, chest, and other areas of the body.

g. Sudden attacks of suffocation at night, forcing the patient to sit up or get out of bed and to gasp for air.

h. Distention of the veins of the neck.

How long does it take a damaged or strained heart to go into failure?

The time required is extremely variable from patient to patient. The heart has an amazing capacity to do its work under great handicaps for a period of many years and will continue to do so provided the obstacles do not become overwhelming.

Once the heart begins to decompensate (fail), does it mean that the patient will die?

No. A decompensating heart may be bolstered for many years with

570

proper care, such as limitation of activity, salt restriction, digitalis therapy, diuretics (drugs that increase the elimination of water and salt by the kidneys), or surgery in specially indicated instances.

How does a physician evaluate the cardiac status of a patient?

    a. By taking a careful history of symptoms and past illnesses.

    b. By listening to the heart through a stethoscope.

    c. By fluoroscoping or x-raying the heart.

    d. By taking an electrocardiogram.

    e. By performing other, more exhaustive tests.

What is an electrocardiogram?

Heart muscle generates a feeble, though characteristic, electrical current when it contracts and relaxes. This current can be picked up

A Patient Having an Electrocardiogram Test Performed.   This is a painless procedure which indicates whether the heart is functioning normally. However, not all heart diseases can be diagnosed through this test.

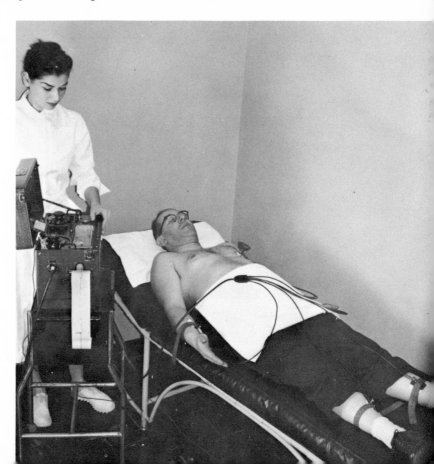

and recorded on paper by a very sensitive instrument known as an electrocardiograph. Variations in amplitude and direction of the current may give important information concerning the heart's function and state of health.

Are electrocardiographic findings in themselves sufficient to establish a patient's cardiac status?

No. They give only supplementary information. The electrocardiogram may be completely normal in the presence of a serious heart disorder. On the other hand, it may demonstrate abnormalities at a time when the physical examination is essentially normal.

What is cardiac catheterization?

There are a number of situations in the evaluation of a patient's heart in which the methods listed above do not yield enough information. In such instances, cardiac catheterization may be performed. This consists of passing and threading a long, narrow, hollow plastic tube into the blood vessel of one of the extremities until it reaches one or more chambers of the heart. Pressure recordings are made through the tube and blood samples are withdrawn. This is not a routine procedure and requires the skill of a specially trained physician. Cardiac catheterization is not usually undertaken unless it is thought that heart surgery may be indicated. (Cardiac catheterization has become an important research tool, adding immensely to our knowledge concerning the working of the heart.)

What is angiocardiography?

Primarily, angiocardiography is used for the same reasons as cardiac catheterization and under similar circumstances. However, it does impart a somewhat different type of information. It consists of injecting into the bloodstream a chemical which is opaque to x-rays. X-rays of the heart are taken in rapid progression as this chemical passes through the various chambers.

This procedure, also, is not employed routinely and requires specialized skills and training. However, in recent years, it has contributed greatly to our knowledge of heart function.

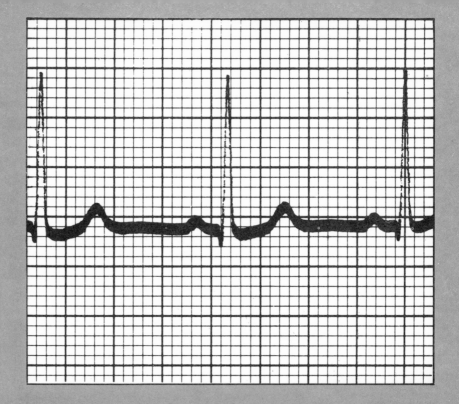

Normal Electrocardiographic Tracing. Cardiologists interpret variations from normal tracings and thereby diagnose heart disease.

Coronary Thrombosis. This electrocardiographic tracing shows that the patient has had an acute coronary thrombosis. It is not difficult to note the variation in this tracing from the normal electrocardiographic tracing shown in the previous illustration.

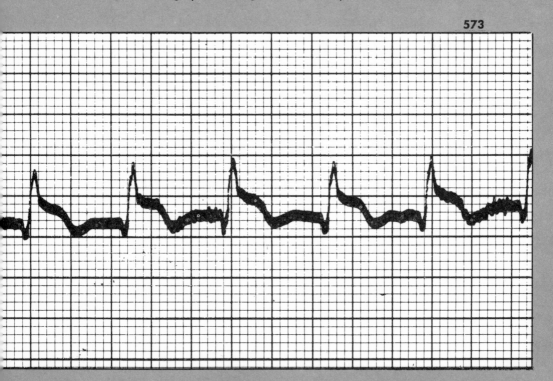

BLOOD PRESSURE

What is blood pressure?

Blood pressure is the force created by the contracting heart in order to keep the blood circulating adequately and constantly through the blood vessels of the body.

In order to overcome the resistance which is present in miles of narrow blood vessels, and in order for the blood to finally arrive at the tissues with enough residual pressure to effect an interchange of chemicals, the heart must maintain a certain minimal level of pressure within the circulatory system.

How is blood pressure measured?

A tubular rubber cuff is strapped around the upper arm. The cuff is connected to an apparatus which measures pressure and it is inflated with air while the physician listens to the arterial pulse in the crook of the elbow. The air pressure in the cuff is raised until the pulsation can no longer be heard. After this, the cuff is deflated until the physician begins to hear the pulse beat return. This is known as the systolic pressure. The cuff is gradually deflated further until the pulse beat again disappears. The pressure at this point is called the diastolic pressure.

What causes high blood pressure?

It is thought that narrowing of the smaller arteries throughout the body causes the heart to pump harder to get the blood to the various tissues. When the heart pumps harder, blood pressure is elevated.

Is there a hereditary tendency toward high blood pressure (essential hypertension)?

Yes, but it should be stated that the presence of high blood pressure in a parent does not necessarily imply that the offspring will have hypertension.

Does overweight tend toward elevated blood pressure?

Yes.

Is high blood pressure caused by eating "red meat," salt, or spices?

No.

Why may high blood pressure be harmful?

a. A greater-than-average strain is placed upon the heart. If it is prolonged, the heart may become enlarged and damaged.

b. Greater wear and tear is placed upon all the blood vessels since blood courses through them at greater pressure. Eventually, vital damage may be inflicted upon these vessels. This, in turn, causes impairment of function of the tissues and organs that they supply. Organs particularly susceptible to such damage are the heart, brain, kidneys, and eyes.

Taking a Blood Pressure Reading. Blood pressure is the force which the heart exerts in pumping the blood through the blood vessels out to the tissues of the body. When blood pressure is high, it means that the heart is pumping with extra force. Prolonged over many years, this serious strain may eventually lead to heart failure.

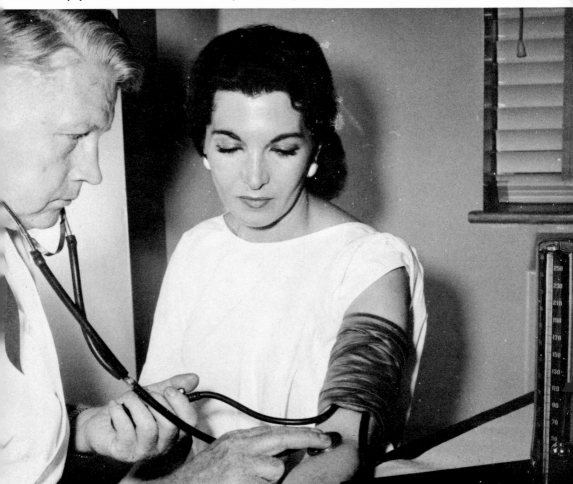

Is there a variation in the way different individuals react to high blood pressure?

Yes. Females are able to withstand continuous high blood pressure levels much better than males. Also, there is a great variation in reaction among different people.

Is high blood pressure curable?

Not really, but modern methods of medication make it possible to keep the pressure under control, thereby minimizing serious potential injury.

In addition to medication and a sensible pattern of living, reduction of overweight and constant surveillance will contribute substantially toward the control of high blood pressure.

On the other hand, there are other, less common causes of hypertension—such as certain tumors, kidney diseases, and endocrine disturbances—which can actually be cured, providing the underlying cause is detectable and can be eradicated.

Can high blood pressure (essential hypertension) be prevented?

No, but the above measures can in many instances lead to its control.

Do emotion and temperament affect the blood pressure?

Yes. Imprudent living and extravagant emotional excesses can raise blood pressure. Such extremes of conduct are thought not to be the basic cause for hypertension but, rather, aggravating influences.

Can a patient with high blood pressure feel healthy and be unaware of its presence?

Many people have high blood pressure for years without being aware of it.

What are the usual symptoms of high blood pressure?

Actually, there are none specifically attributable to the elevated pressure. The headaches and hot flashes complained about are usually due to other conditions.

What is the normal blood pressure level?

There is no such thing as a set, normal blood pressure. There is a wide range of pressures considered normal for the average adult. The upper limit of normal systolic pressure is about 150 to 160 millimeters of mercury, and the upper limit for the diastolic pressure is from ninety to one hundred.

What is low blood pressure?

The common or garden variety of low blood pressure is not a disease. It refers to a state in which blood pressure readings are found to be in the lower level of the normal range. This is usually a healthy situation, for it means that the heart and blood vessels are not being put to undue strain.

Is low blood pressure ever an evidence of true disease?

In certain rare diseases, persistent low blood pressure is found as a constant sign.

Does the common form of low blood pressure give rise to symptoms such as fatigue or lethargy?

Only rarely. Unfortunately, low blood pressure has become a psychological hatrack upon which many individuals hang a variety of unrelated complaints.

Does low blood pressure require treatment?

Rarely, if ever.

Can one have "temporary" high blood pressure?

Yes. Often the excitement of an examination or the circumstances surrounding an examination may give rise to abnormally high pressure readings. Later examination under more relaxed conditions may yield a perfectly normal result. Also, exceptional emotional stress may cause elevated blood pressure for a period of several days or weeks. This will usually return to normal when the strain is eased.

CONGENITAL HEART DISEASE

What types of congenital heart conditions are there?

a. Abnormal communications between the right and left sides of the heart, so that blood from the veins passes into the arterial circulation.

b. Abnormalities in the structure and function of the heart valves which separate the various chambers of the heart.

c. Abnormalities in the heart muscle itself.

d. Abnormalities in the inner and outer linings of the heart.

What causes congenital heart conditions?

Defects in prenatal development.

Are congenital heart conditions hereditary?

No.

Can abnormalities of the heart be detected immediately after the child is born?

Some may be detected by listening with a stethoscope at birth or noting the blue color of the baby. Other conditions remain obscure until much later in childhood or even until adulthood.

How common are congenital heart conditions?

They occur approximately three times in every thousand births.

Are congenital heart conditions serious?

Yes, because they often lead to impairment of heart function and circulation, and produce situations in which the tissues receive an insufficient quantity of oxygen.

What is a "blue baby"?

A baby born with a condition in which oxygen-poor blood from the veins passes directly from the right side of the circulatory system to the left or arterial side. This blood by-passes the lungs and is therefore deficient in oxygen.

Can congenital heart abnormalities be cured?

In the past few years tremendous strides have been made surgically in the treatment of these conditions. Some abnormalities can be cured completely through surgery, others may be helped considerably. (See the section on Heart Surgery in this chapter.)

CORONARY ARTERY DISEASE

What are the coronary arteries?

They are the blood vessels which course through the wall of the heart and nourish the heart muscle. They are the first blood vessels to branch off from the aorta as it leaves the heart.

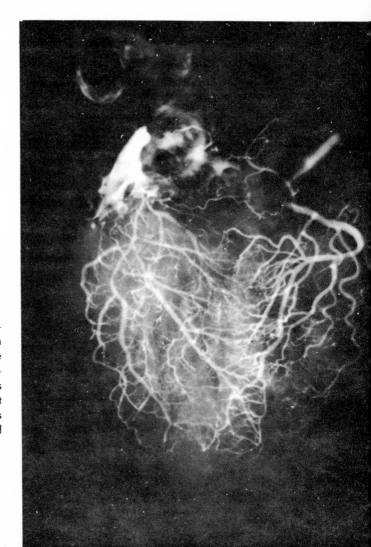

The Coronary Arteries. This illustration shows a heart specimen in which the coronary arteries have been injected with dye. It demonstrates that the coronary arteries supply blood to the wall of the heart itself. Blockage of these arteries causes serious heart damage and may result in sudden death.

What is coronary artery disease?

Since the heart muscle expends a huge amount of energy in its cease-less work, it naturally demands a good supply of blood. Any impairment of these blood vessels that interferes with adequate blood flow is known as coronary artery disease.

What is the most frequent cause of coronary artery disease?

Arteriosclerosis (hardening of the arteries).

What is coronary insufficiency and angina pectoris?

If the blood flow through the coronary arteries is significantly diminished, the heart cannot function at maximum efficiency. The heart then signals its plight by registering pain or discomfort in the chest—usually under the breastbone. Often, however, the discomfort or pain may be manifest in more remote regions of the body, such as in the back, arms, neck, jaw, or upper abdomen. The registering of such pain, with or without exertion, is called angina pectoris. The pain subsides when the patient rests and stops any physical exertion.

What is coronary occlusion?

It is the complete interruption of blood flow through one of the branches of the coronary artery. As a result, a portion of heart muscle may be destroyed from lack of nourishment. This is called myocardial infarction. If a large main artery is blocked, a large portion of heart muscle is damaged. If a small subsidiary branch is blocked, a smaller portion of muscle is damaged. The term "heart attack" is commonly used to allude to this sequence of events.

What is the cause of coronary occlusion?

The most common cause is the blockage of the coronary arteries by the formation of a blood clot. This is termed coronary thrombosis. It usually occurs at a site where the artery was previously damaged by arteriosclerosis.

What are some of the factors which govern the outcome of a heart attack?

a. The amount of previous heart damage.

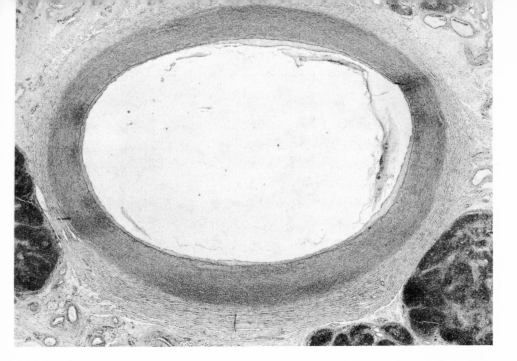

Normal Coronary Artery. This photomicrograph shows a cross-section of a normal coronary artery. Note how wide and open is the passageway in the middle of the vessel.

Coronary Thrombosis. This photomicrograph shows a cross-section of an arteriosclerotic coronary artery in which thrombosis (a clot) has taken place. Naturally, no blood can flow through such an artery and the heart muscle wall supplied by such an artery will be severely damaged from lack of circulation.

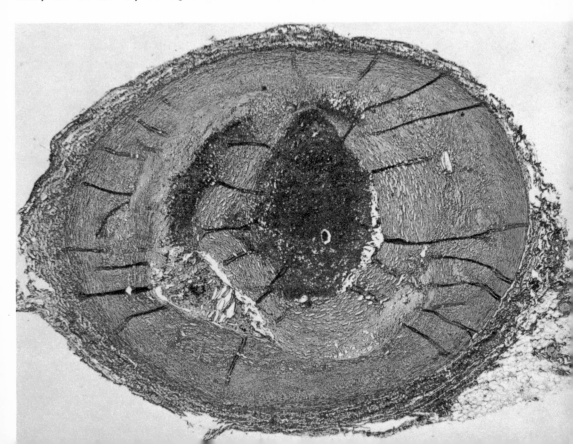

b. The size of the area of heart muscle damaged by the particular attack.

c. The amount of remaining normal heart muscle.

d. The degree to which the coronary obstruction spreads toward other branches of the artery.

e. The occurrence or absence of disorders in the rhythm of the heart.

f. The presence or absence of blood clots on the inner wall of the heart that may break off and travel to other parts of the body.

g. The possibility of rupture of the weakened heart wall.

What are the chances of recovery from an initial coronary thrombosis?

Approximately nineteen out of twenty people will recover from their initial attack.

What is the significance of coronary insufficiency or angina pectoris?

Angina pectoris is a term applied to the chest pain caused by coronary insufficiency. There are many degrees of angina pectoris and many degrees of coronary insufficiency. Mild degrees are compatible with all but the most strenuous activity. Severe degrees may completely incapacitate a patient.

Do all people with angina pectoris eventually develop coronary occlusion?

No, though it is true that such patients are definitely more prone to such heart attacks.

Is angina pectoris compatible with a normal life span?

Yes. However, the individual outlook depends on many factors that vary from patient to patient.

Can attacks of angina pectoris be prevented?

To a certain extent; that is, a more orderly, regulated life with the deletion of excessive work and excitement, plus the taking of certain medications, may control attacks of angina pectoris. In some cases, they can be avoided completely.

Is surgery helpful in coronary artery disease?

A number of surgical procedures have been devised to improve blood flow to heart muscle, but this field of surgery is still too new to be definitely evaluated. However, it is reasonable to assume that real and solid advances will be made in this direction in the not-too-distant future.

What is the treatment for coronary occlusion (thrombosis)?

The mainstay of treatment is bed rest in the early stages, and limited activity for a prolonged period afterward. Anticoagulant drugs may be given to prevent further spread of the blood clot. Medications to relieve pain are also of considerable benefit.

Why are bed rest and limited physical activity important?

The less active the individual, the less the heart has to work to supply the necessary circulatory support. It may not seem so, but there is a tremendous difference in the amount of energy expended by the heart during absolute rest and ordinary activity.

How long must a patient with a coronary occlusion stay in bed?

This depends upon the extent and progress of the illness. On the average, a patient with a heart attack may be required to stay in bed from three to six weeks.

How long must a patient who has had a coronary occlusion stop working?

On the average, most patients may return to work three months after the onset. It is wise that these people increase their activity in a gradual fashion, rather than "plunge right in." It is also important that the patient provide for modification in his occupation if it is unduly taxing. Most patients who have had a heart attack *can* and *should* return to work, but they must avoid emotional as well as physical strain.

What percentage of people who have had coronary thrombosis can make a good recovery and return to work?

Statistics show that four out of five patients who have had a heart attack make an excellent recovery and return to their usual occupation.

Can a patient who has had a "heart attack" look forward to many years of life?

Yes. Patients who have had serious heart attacks often live twenty-five to thirty or more years thereafter.

What are anticoagulant drugs?

They are chemical compounds which decrease the normal clotting ability of the blood. (Heparin and dicumarol are two of the most frequently used.)

Why are anticoagulant drugs used in treating coronary thrombosis?

a. To prevent the clot in the artery from spreading, thus further impairing the blood supply to the heart muscle.

b. To prevent clots from forming on the inner lining of the heart and in the leg veins, since the clots may break loose and travel in the bloodstream (embolism).

Is it possible to predict the onset of a heart attack?

Not always. It often occurs without warning to people who have been in apparent good health and who may have had a normal electrocardiogram just prior to the attack. There are instances, however, where warning signs—such as chest pains—may have occurred for weeks or months prior to an acute attack.

Can periodic electrocardiograms give advance information as to the possibility of a future heart attack?

Only to a very limited extent.

What age group is most susceptible to a heart attack?

People between forty and sixty years of age.

Are men more susceptible to heart attack than women?

Yes. They are approximately three times more prone to coronary artery disease.

Is there a hereditary susceptibility to coronary artery disease?

There sometimes appears to be a hereditary predisposition, but this is not an exclusive determining factor in the causation of the disease.

What influence does physical exertion have upon the immediate or future occurrence of coronary heart disease?

Generally speaking, physical exertion is not a highly significant factor in the cause of heart attacks. However, there have been instances of heart attacks having occurred concomitantly with, or shortly after, severe physical exertion. The consensus is that most of these people had quiescent underlying disease of the coronary arteries which predisposed them to attacks.

How important is emotional strain in the production of a heart attack?

It is thought to be a contributing factor although it is usually not the sole or the main causative agent.

What abnormal conditions predispose one toward the development of coronary artery disease?

The two most common disorders which increase a patient's susceptibility to coronary artery disease are diabetes and high blood pressure.

What is the influence of diet on coronary artery disease?

All physicians are agreed that it is important to avoid overweight. It is probably important to keep the ingestion of fatty foods down to a minimum.

What is the influence of smoking upon coronary artery disease?

In some people, smoking causes spasm of the coronary artery. It is therefore injurious and should be stopped by those who have a tendency toward coronary insufficiency.

HEART IRREGULARITIES
(Cardiac Arrhythmia)

What is cardiac arrhythmia?

An irregularity in the rhythmic beat of the heart.

585

What causes cardiac irregularity?

Some cases are caused by true heart disease; others are associated with normal hearts which for one reason or another go "off beat." The physician can usually distinguish between the various causes for such irregularities.

Do irregularities of the heart interfere with its function?

An occasional extra beat or skip (extrasystole) has little effect upon heart function. Other cardiac arrhythmias may seriously interfere with circulation.

Can cardiac irregularities be treated successfully?

In the great majority of cases, cardiac irregularities will respond to treatment with certain heart drugs.

What is a skipped beat or premature beat?

This is an occasional irregularity of the heart in which the patient is aware of a peculiar sensation ("butterfly") in the chest or a fleeting, sinking, or empty sensation in the chest. Technically, it is known as an extrasystole.

What is the significance of a skipped beat?

In the vast majority of cases, there is no serious significance to this, although at times it may be annoying.

What causes skipped beats?

A variety of conditions, among which are exhaustion, the unwise taking of drugs, nervousness, irritability, an acute infection, etc. Less commonly, the cause may be underlying heart disease.

Is the use of tobacco ever a cause for extrasystoles?

Yes, this is one of the commonest causes for cardiac irregularity.

ATHLETE'S HEART

What is "athlete's heart"?

This term has been used erroneously in most instances to refer to enlargement of the heart in people who had overexerted themselves during days of strenuous athletics. At present, it is felt that these hearts were, in effect, basically unsound to begin with. There is no sure evidence that indulgence in athletics produces heart disease in a normal heart.

PALPITATION OF THE HEART

What is meant by "palpitation of the heart"?

This is a non-medical expression often used to denote consciousness of a rapid and exceptionally forceful heartbeat. Occasionally, this feeling of palpitation is associated with irregularities of the heartbeat.

Does palpitation denote heart disease?

Usually not. It occurs most often in people who are suffering from undue tension and anxiety.

PAROXYSMAL ARRHYTHMIA

What is paroxysmal arrhythmia?

This is a condition in which the heart suddenly and abruptly goes into another rhythm, often becoming extremely rapid. These attacks may come on suddenly, at frequent or infrequent intervals, without warning.

How long do attacks of paroxysmal arrhythmia last?

Anywhere from a few minutes to a few days.

Do these attacks occur only in diseased hearts?

No. Often, the heart is completely normal.

What causes episodes of paroxysmal arrhythmia?

a. In organic heart conditions, it is usually a disease of the "rhythm centers."

b. In normal hearts, the cause is usually unknown.

HEART BLOCK

What is heart block?

A condition in which the electrical impulse from the atrium of the heart is not transmitted normally to the ventricle.

Is heart block usually associated with a disease of the heart?

Yes.

How is the diagnosis of heart block usually made?

By noting the abnormality on the electrocardiographic tracing.

Is heart block compatible with life?

Yes. Many people with heart block can live comfortably for long periods of time.

FIBRILLATION OF THE HEART

What is auricular fibrillation?

It is a condition in which there is complete disorder, originating in the auricles, in the rhythmic beat of the heart.

What causes auricular fibrillation?

It is commonly seen in long-standing rheumatic heart disease, arteriosclerotic heart disease, and in hyperthyroidism (a disease in which there is overactivity of the thyroid gland).

What is the significance of auricular fibrillation?

An irregularly beating heart is usually not as efficient as one that beats regularly, and it therefore pumps blood to the tissues in an inefficient manner.

What complications may occur with chronic auricular fibrillation of the heart?

a. Because of too rapid and irregular contractions, the output of the heart may be inadequate and may lead to heart failure or decompensation.

b. A fibrillating heart may develop clots of blood on its inner wall. If these should break off and travel to other organs of the body, they can cause severe damage (embolization).

Can a fibrillating heart be brought back to normal rhythm?

In many instances, this can be accomplished and maintained. Patients with a fibrillating heart may be placed upon medications for many weeks or months. In other instances, the condition becomes permament.

HEART MURMURS

What is a heart murmur?

An abnormal sound produced by the beating heart.

How can a physician make a diagnosis of a heart murmur?

By listening with a stethoscope.

Do heart murmurs cause symptoms?

No. The patient is usually unaware that a murmur exists.

Do all murmurs indicate heart disease?

No. A high percentage of murmurs are produced by normal hearts and are of no clinical significance.

What is a functional heart murmur?

One not associated with heart disease.

What is an organic murmur?

A murmur that is associated with heart disease.

Can a doctor tell the difference between an organic and a functional murmur?

Usually, it is quite simple for the physician to determine the difference by the location and position of the murmur, by the heartbeat cycle, and by other distinctive features.
A small percentage of murmurs remain in question and diagnosis is quite difficult.

HEART VALVE INFECTION
(Bacterial Endocarditis)

What is bacterial endocarditis?

Heart valves previously damaged by rheumatic fever, congenital heart disease, or other pathology, are particularly susceptible to bacterial infection. This is called bacterial endocarditis. This complication is an extremely serious one and, unless promptly treated, causes irreparable destruction of the valves. In addition, bacteria are carried by the bloodstream to other organs of the body, which in turn may also be seriously damaged.

Is bacterial endocarditis curable?

At the present time successful treatment is available for the majority of these cases.

What is the treatment for bacterial endocarditis?

The prolonged and intensive administration of antibiotics.

Is bacterial endocarditis preventable?

To a degree, yes. Any infection in the body should be promptly and vigorously treated, lest bacteria break through the tissue barriers and enter the bloodstream to become implanted upon a heart valve.

What other measures should be taken to prevent the onset of bacterial endocarditis?

All people suffering from rheumatic heart disease should be particularly careful about surgical procedures. For instance, the extraction of a tooth should be preceded and followed by antibiotic therapy.

HEART SURGERY

What conditions can be helped through heart surgery?

a. Congenital heart conditions:
  1. Patent ductus arteriosus, the persistence of a blood vessel which ordinarily closes by the time the child is born.

2. Septal defects—abnormal opening and connections between the various chambers of the heart.

3. The condition that causes blue babies—abnormal position and connections of major blood vessels leading to and from the heart.

4. Pulmonic stenosis, a condition in which there is either an underdeveloped pulmonary artery leading from the heart to the lungs, or a constricted pulmonary valve opening.

5. Coarctation of the aorta, a narrowing of the aorta in the chest.

b. Acquired heart conditions:

1. Rheumatic heart disease, a condition in which there is constriction or other deformity of the heart valves secondary to rheumatic fever.

c. Coronary artery disease.

d. Pericarditis, an inflammatory condition of the sheath (pericardium) which surrounds the heart.

e. Heart injuries:

1. Stab wounds or gunshot wounds.

2. Aneurysm of the heart, in which there is a bulge of the muscle wall secondary to damage caused by a previous coronary thrombosis.

Are operations upon the heart dangerous?

Refinements in the techniques have reduced the dangers of heart surgery remarkably, so that it is fast approaching the degree of safety obtained in some of the other major fields of surgical endeavor.

Can all people with heart disease be operated upon?

No. Only certain types of heart conditions lend themselves to surgical help.

Is it difficult to approach the heart surgically?

No. Incisions into the chest cavity make the heart readily available to the surgeon.

591

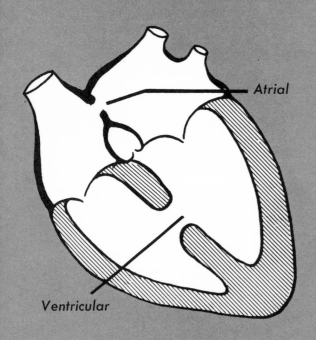

Atrial

Ventricular

Septal Defects. This diagram shows defects in the walls between the various heart chambers. Newer advances in heart surgery have made it possible to open the heart and repair septal defects. During the operation the patient's circulation is conducted with the help of a heart pump, so that the heart is bypassed until the surgical repair is completed.

HEART DEFECTS WHICH CAN BE CORRECTED SURGICALLY

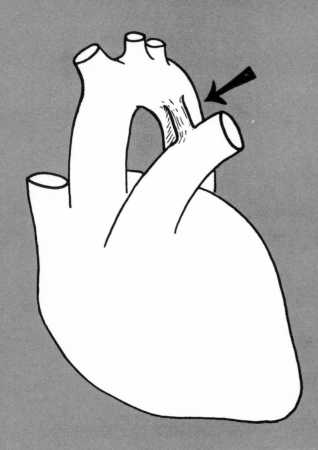

Patent Ductus Arteriosus. This diagram shows a common congenital heart deformity known as patent ductus arteriosus. This can be corrected surgically by tying off the artery. People born with this abnormality can now be cured by a simple, safe heart operation.

Mitral Stenosis. This illustration shows one of the most common of all heart conditions, mitral stenosis. This disease is characterized by a narrowing of the valve between the left atrium and the left ventricle of the heart. Mitral stenosis is the end result of a severe attack of rheumatic fever.

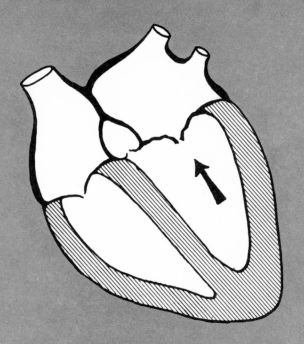

HEART DEFECTS WHICH CAN BE CORRECTED SURGICALLY

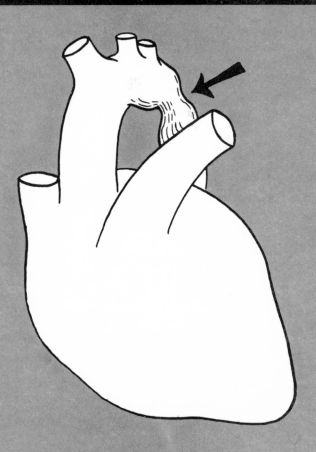

Coarctation of Aorta. This diagram shows a birth deformity of the vessels of the heart known as coarctation of the aorta. With newer surgical techniques, it is now possible to remove this constricted portion of the aorta and to reshape it to allow for normal circulation.

593

How successful are heart operations for congenital defects?

Almost all of those suffering from a patent ductus arteriosus can be cured; approximately 85 to 90 per cent of those with coarctation of the aorta can be cured; and approximately 75 per cent of the blue babies can be cured. Recent advances in the approach to septal defects, utilizing various heart pumps and open heart surgery, augur well for the curability of this type of deformity in the near future.

Can patients with congenital heart defects, successfully operated upon, look forward to a more normal life?

Yes. Many children who were labeled heart cripples can now look forward to near-normal lives after heart surgery.

Do congenital defects often come back once they have been corrected?

No.

Is surgery for rheumatic heart disease successful?

Yes. The great majority of those who have constriction of the mitral or aortic valves can be helped tremendously through surgery.

What percentage survive of those operated upon for rheumatic heart disease?

Approximately 90 to 95 per cent.

What percentage are benefited by such surgery?

Almost all of those who are operated upon.

Do all patients with rheumatic heart disease require surgery?

No. Surgery is limited to those whose lives are severely handicapped by the disease.

Is life expectancy improved by operations upon hearts which have been affected by rheumatic fever?

Yes.

Do these patients often return to normal living?

Yes.

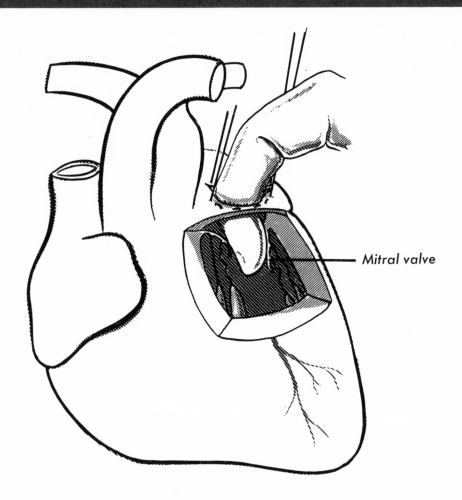

Mitral valve

Operation to Relieve Mitral Stenosis. In this operation, called mitral commissurotomy, the surgeon inserts his finger into the heart (left atrium) to break adhesions of the deformed, narrowed valve. By inserting a specially designed knife, he may also cut some of the constricted valve, thus allowing a more normal blood flow. Newer surgical methods involve repair of the damaged valve under direct vision with the heart opened. Mitral commissurotomy is followed by relief of the condition in the vast majority of cases.

What operations are performed upon those with coronary artery disease?

Several operations have been devised. The most popular one today is called poudrage.

What is a poudrage operation?

It is the instillation of talcum powder into the pericardium (lining membrane around the heart).

How does poudrage help a patient with angina pectoris or coronary artery disease?

The talcum powder is said to produce an inflammation which, in turn, results in the formation of new blood vessels. Thus, there is an increased circulation to the wall of the heart.

Does poudrage appear to be the final answer to surgical help in coronary artery disease?

No. Much new investigative work is presently being undertaken in this field.

What newer operations are being done for coronary artery disease?

Various operations for the improvement of circulation to the heart muscle, such as the transplantation of vessels into the heart muscle wall. Also, attempts are being made to restitute the narrowed channels of the existing coronary arteries by coring them out.

What anesthesia is used for heart operations?

An inhalation anesthesia given through a tube placed in the trachea.

Where is the incision made for heart operations?

Between the ribs that overlie the left side of the chest.

Have methods been devised which permit by-passing of the heart during surgery?

Yes, there are heart pumps which can take the place of the heart during the time that it is undergoing surgery. This permits the surgeon to open the heart and operate upon it under direct vision and in a bloodless field.

What is meant by "hypothermia" in heart surgery?

This means freezing the patient's body so that his heart action is slowed down markedly. This permits the surgeon to work upon the heart while it is more at rest and when blood flow is greatly curtailed.

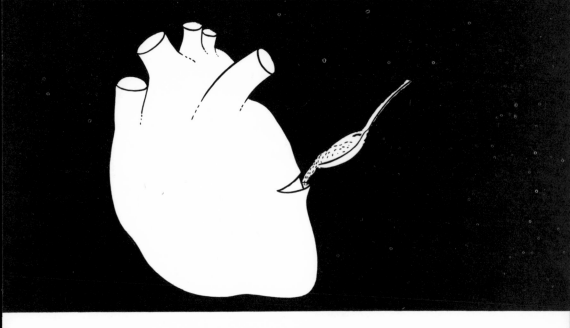

Poudrage. This operation involves the placing of sterile talc powder into the sac (pericardium) surrounding the heart in order to improve the blood supply to the heart muscle wall. People who suffer from angina pectoris (attacks of pain in the heart area) are sometimes benefited by this operative procedure.

When will physicians recommend heart surgery?

a. When it is felt that the ultimate chances for survival are greater with surgery than without surgery.

b. When a person is leading an invalided, useless life, and desires the chance for more normal living through heart surgery.

c. When a reasonable chance for cure or improvement exists through heart surgery and when the patient or his family fully understand the risks involved.

Are heart operations lengthy?

Yes. Some heart operations take several hours to perform.

Are heart operations painful?

No. Patients are usually quite comfortable during recovery from a heart operation.

Do heart conditions tend to recur once they have been benefited by heart surgery?

No. The majority of successful results in heart surgery are of a permanent nature.

27 *Hernia*

What is a hernia?

A hernia is a defect in a body compartment (cavity) which permits a structure to leave its normal confines and to extend into a region where it does not belong. As an example, in a hernia of the diaphragm, the stomach may leave the abdominal cavity and enter the chest cavity through the diaphragmatic defect.

What other name is used for hernia?

The word "rupture" is frequently used to denote a hernia.

What causes hernia?

The great majority of hernias are caused by defects or weakness in the muscular and connective tissue structures which separate the various compartments or cavities of the body, such as the chest from the abdomen, or the abdomen from the limbs. Other hernias result from an injury which tears the muscular or connective tissue barriers at various exit points of the body compartments.

Are many hernias present at birth?

Yes. A sizable number of children are born with hernias because of defects in development. These are commonly noted in the region of the navel (umbilical hernia) or in the groin (inguinal hernia).

At what specific areas in the body are hernias most likely to occur?

At the various points where large structures, such as blood vessels or portions of the intestinal tract, leave or enter the various body cavities. At these sites there are loose tissues which, when placed under great strain, may separate and tear.

What types of strain or injury are most likely to lead to a rupture?

a. Lifting of heavy objects.

b. Sudden twists, pulls, or muscle strains.

c. Marked gains in weight which cause an increase in intra-abdominal pressure.

d. The growth of a large abdominal tumor which displaces the organs.

e. Pregnancy, with its accompanying increase in intra-abdominal pressure.

f. Chronic constipation, with its associated straining at stool.

g. Repeated attacks of coughing which create sudden increases in intra-abdominal pressure.

How common is hernia?

It is one of the most common of all conditions requiring surgery.

Are men more prone than women to develop hernia?

Yes, if it is the type which results from physical strain and effort, such as hernia in the groin (inguinal hernia). Women are more likely to get hernias of the umbilical region (navel) as a result of pregnancy.

Do hernias tend to run in families or to be inherited?

No, but the kind of muscular development that one possesses does tend to be inherited.

What are the most common types of hernia?

a. Inguinal hernia. This is the most prevalent type of hernia. It occurs in the groin, often developing on both sides of the body. Such ruptures are called bilateral inguinal hernias.

599

b. Femoral hernia. This type is located just below the groin and occurs alongside the large blood vessels which extend from the trunk into the lower limbs.

c. Ventral hernia. This type usually occurs in the midline of the abdomen below the navel, and often takes place as a result of the separation of the muscles of the abdominal wall following pregnancy.

d. Epigastric hernia. This type is located in the upper midline of the abdomen above the navel. Such hernias probably exist from birth but only become apparent in adult life.

e. Umbilical hernia. This is one of the most common forms of hernia and takes place in the region of the navel. Newborns and women who have had many pregnancies appear to be particularly prone to develop umbilical hernias.

f. Incisional hernia. This type of hernia occurs through an operative scar, either because of poor healing power of the wound or because infection has caused the tissues to heal inadequately. A hernia of this type can be located anywhere on the abdominal wall.

g. Recurrent hernia. About one in ten hernias will recur after surgical repair. This is called recurrent hernia.

h. Diaphragmatic hernia. This is an extremely common defect and takes place most frequently alongside the point where the esophagus (food pipe) passes through the diaphragm from the chest into the abdomen. Other diaphragmatic hernias result from lack of development of the diaphragm or from rupture of the diaphragm due to an injury. These hernias are characterized by abdominal organs—such as a portion of stomach, small intestine, or large bowel—entering the defect and lodging in the chest cavity.

i. Internal hernia. This is an unusual type of rupture in which an internal abdominal organ, usually the small intestine, enters crevices or subdivisions of the abdominal cavity, where it does not belong.

j. Gluteal and lumbar hernia. These hernias are extremely rare and are due to defects in the musculature of the buttocks or back.

Direct Inguinal Hernia

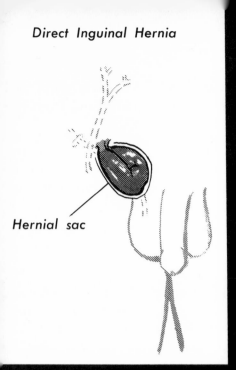

Hernial sac

Indirect Inguinal Hernia

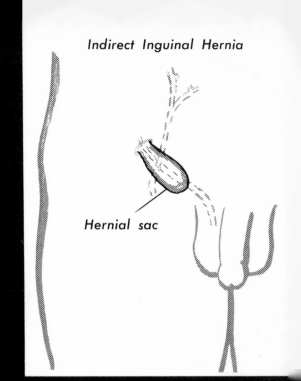

Hernial sac

Sliding Inguinal Hernia

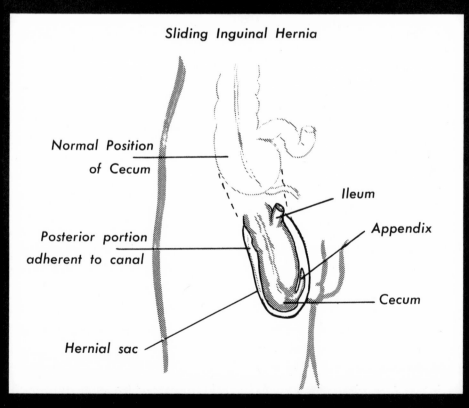

Normal Position
of Cecum

Ileum

Appendix

Posterior portion
adherent to canal

Cecum

Hernial sac

nguinal Hernia.   The accompanying diagrams show various types of inguinal herniae,
r hernias which are located in the groin. If the patient is in satisfactory general health,
urgery should be performed for their repair. Failure to undergo surgery may result in
loop of bowel becoming caught within the hernial sac thus producing bowel strangula-

UMBILICAL HERNIA

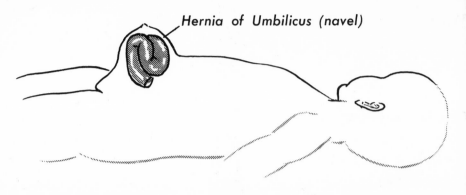

Hernia of Umbilicus (navel)

Umbilical Hernia or Hernia of the Navel. Many children are born with small umbilical hernias. The majority of these will heal by themselves within the first year of life. If the hernia persists, it is advisable to have it repaired surgically. The operation for repair of an umbilical hernia is a simple, safe procedure.

The herniated organs will appear as bulges posteriorly in either the buttocks or the back.

When is medical, rather than surgical, management advocated in the treatment of hernia?

  a. If a hernia has recurred two or more times after surgery and the patient's tissue structures appear to be poor, it is probably best not to attempt surgical repair a third or fourth time, as it will be met with failure in a large percentage of cases.

  b. People who are markedly overweight should not be operated upon until they reduce, as repairs in these people are notoriously unsuccessful.

  c. People with serious medical conditions, such as active tuberculosis or serious heart disease, are probably best treated without surgery.

  d. People with small hernias who are in their seventh or eighth decade of life are perhaps best treated medically unless the hernia causes severe symptoms.

What is the medical treatment for hernia?

The wearing of a support or truss to hold the hernial contents within the abdominal cavity.

As a general rule, should trusses be worn for prolonged periods of time before surgery is carried out?

No. Trusses tend to weaken the structures with which they are in constant contact. Therefore, they should not be worn for more than a few weeks prior to surgery.

Why isn't the wearing of a truss advised rather than surgery, in all hernias?

Because trusses do not cure hernias. They merely hold the hernial contents in place. As people get older and hernias enlarge, trusses work less satisfactorily.

Are any dangers involved in neglecting to operate upon hernias?

Definitely, yes. The chance of strangulation of bowel is always present, and such a situation is dangerous to life.

Is the injection treatment satisfactory in the treatment of hernias?

No. This method has been abandoned as dangerous and ineffectual.

Do hernias tend to disappear by themselves?

No. The only hernias which ever disappear by themselves are the small hernias of the navel seen in newborns, and an occasional small inguinal hernia in a newborn.

How effective is surgery in the treatment of hernia?

The vast majority of hernias can be repaired successfully by restoring and reinforcing the torn structures, replacing the extruded structures into their normal anatomical location, and by removing the outpouching of abdominal tissue (peritoneum) which makes up the hernial sac.

When is the best time to operate upon hernias?

Hernia operations are usually elective procedures and the time for

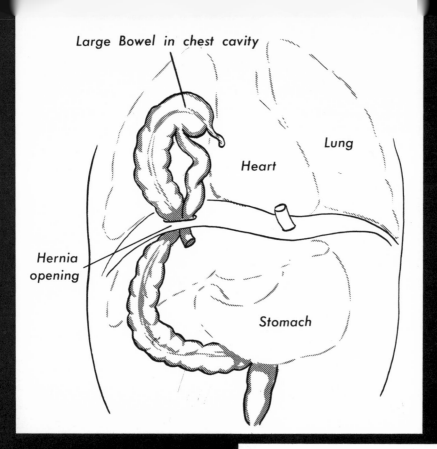

Large Bowel in chest cavity

Lung

Heart

Hernia opening

Stomach

DIAPHRAGMATIC HERNIAS

Hernia of the Diaphragm, with Organs from the Abdomen Ascending into the Chest Cavity. This is a serious type of hernia but it can be repaired effectively by surgery. In most cases the surgery is performed by opening the chest cavity and closing the hole in the diaphragm from above. A popular term for a diaphragmatic hernia is "upside-down stomach."

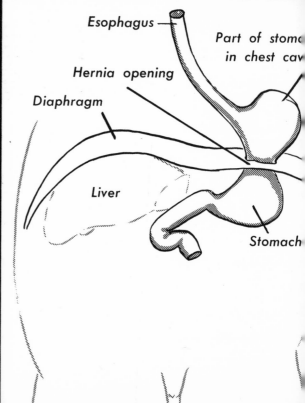

Esophagus

Part of stomach in chest cavity

Hernia opening

Diaphragm

Liver

Stomach

their repair can be chosen by the patient to suit his convenience. It must be remembered, however, that most hernias tend to enlarge; the larger the hernia, the more difficult it is to repair and the greater the chance of subsequent recurrence.

When is a hernia operation an emergency procedure?

When the hernia strangulates, a condition in which an organ, such as the intestine or bowel, is caught in the hernial sac and its blood supply is interfered with. Under such circumstances, the patient must be operated upon immediately! Failure to do so will lead to gangrene of the strangulated hernial contents and possible death from peritonitis.

Will surgeons delay operations in elective cases if the patient is overweight?

Yes. If the patient is too stout, the repair of the hernia is similar to an attempt at stuffing too much clothing into a small valise. If such a valise does close, the great pressure from within is likely to pop it open!

Are hernia operations dangerous?

No. They are rarely followed by complications, except when the operation has been carried out for strangulation. In such cases, gangrenous bowel or intestine may be encountered, and this will entail extensive serious surgery for removal of the gangrenous portions.

What procedure is carried out when gangrenous intestine or bowel is found in a hernia?

The gangrenous portions of bowel are removed. This is a most serious and complicated operation, with many dangers. The mortality rate in these cases has been lowered remarkably by improved surgical techniques and the use of antibiotic drugs, but the procedure still constitutes one of the most formidable in abdominal surgery.

Are hernia operations particularly painful?

No, except for pain in the operative region for a few days after the surgery has been performed.

Are operations for diaphragmatic hernia particularly dangerous?

No, but these are more extensive procedures than those for hernia's in the abdominal region.

How are diaphragmatic hernias repaired?

In most instances, an incision is made in the chest along the ribs, the chest cavity is opened, and the defect or rent in the diaphragm is sutured after the misplaced organs have been replaced into the abdominal cavity. Another effective approach to this type of repair is through an abdominal incision.

Is repair of a diaphragmatic hernia usually successful?

Yes, in the great majority of cases.

How long do hernia operations take to perform?

The simple inguinal hernias can be repaired in one-half to three-quarters of an hour. The more extensive hernias, such as the diaphragmatic or the incarcerated ones in which the herniated organs are firmly attached to the sac wall, may take several hours to repair.

What kind of anesthesia is used?

For hernias below the level of the navel, spinal anesthesia is most often employed. Diaphragmatic hernias and hernias in the upper abdomen are often operated upon under general inhalation anesthesia.

How long a hospital stay is necessary after surgery?

Six to seven days for the ordinary hernia; ten to twelve days for the more complicated types.

How soon after operation can the patient get out of bed?

With the almost universal employment of early ambulation, most patients get out of bed the day following surgery.

Can coughing or sneezing cause a recurrence of the hernia?

No, despite the fact that patients often feel as though they have ripped open all of their stitches when they cough.

What are the chances of recurrence following surgery?

More than 90 per cent of hernias are cured permanently after surgery. Most recurrences are seen in elderly people or in those who have particularly fragile muscle and connective tissues.

How long does it take for the average hernia wound to heal?

Seven to ten days.

What precautions should be taken to prevent hernia recurrence?

a. The patient should not permit himself to gain a large amount of weight.
b. Pushing, pulling, or lifting heavy objects (those over forty to fifty pounds) should be avoided whenever possible.
c. All strenuous exercise should be avoided for a period of four to six months.

If hernias do recur, what procedure is indicated?

About four out of five recurrent hernias can be cured by reoperation.

Should patients who have been operated upon for hernia wear trusses or abdominal supports?

No. Surgical repair is sufficient protection.

Is it common for patients to have slight pain, numbness, or tingling in the wound or along the scrotum for several weeks or months after hernia operations?

Yes. This happens occasionally but will disappear spontaneously.

Is sex life affected by the repair of an inguinal hernia?

No. The testicles and the other genital structures are not interfered with when hernia repair is carried out.

How soon after birth can an infant have a hernia repaired?

Newborns withstand surgery exceptionally well. If the hernia is large or if there is a danger of bowel strangulation, it is preferable to operate upon these children during the first few weeks or months of life.

Do hernias in the newborn tend to occur in both groins?

Yes. It is becoming the widespread practice to operate upon both sides in these children, even though a hernia may be felt on only one side. Three out of four infants who have a hernia on one side will also have one on the other, though the second hernia may not be discovered on physical examination.

Will operating on both sides increase the risk of surgery?

No.

Can normal physical activity ever be resumed by someone who has undergone a hernia repair?

Most certainly, yes!

Can a woman permit herself to become pregnant after a hernia operation?

Yes, within a few months after surgical recovery.

How soon after a hernia operation can one do the following:

Bathe	Ten to fourteen days.
Walk out on the street	Seven to ten days.
Walk up and down stairs	Seven to ten days.
Perform household duties	Three to four weeks.
Drive a car	Five to six weeks.
Resume marital relations	Four weeks.
Return to work	Six to eight weeks.
Resume all physical activities	Three to six months.

How often should one return for a checkup following a hernia operation?

Approximately every six months, for a period of two years.

28 *Immunizations and Vaccinations*

What is active immunity?

It is the protection afforded by having the disease or by receiving an injection of a substance which stimulates the body to produce long-lasting protective antibodies.

What diseases afford permanent immunity after one has had them?

Measles, scarlet fever, diphtheria, German measles, mumps, chicken pox, and whooping cough. Typhoid fever, smallpox, and poliomyelitis also give permanent immunity if one has had them.

What is meant by passive or inherited immunity?

This is the type of immunity one inherits at birth if the mother has had the disease some time previously. The immunity is passed through the placenta and into the child's bloodstream. Passive immunity can also be accomplished by the injection of convalescent serum from someone who has just recently had the disease, or by the injection of gamma globulin.

Against which diseases are gamma globulin injections effective?

Measles, German measles, infectious hepatitis, and poliomyelitis. Unfortunately, the immunity lasts for only a few weeks.

How long does passive or inherited immunity usually last?

About three to six months. In some instances, as long as nine months.

What is the reason for creating passive immunity if it lasts for only a short time?

It will tide the patient over a period when an epidemic may be in progress and thus spare him from contracting the disease.

Against which diseases is convalescent serum effective?

Mumps, scarlet fever, chicken pox, whooping cough.

Are convalescent serums useful in *treatment* of contagious diseases?

In general, no. However, convalescent serum does have some effectiveness in the treatment of whooping cough.

What is the best immunization schedule for infants?

It is best to give the triple vaccine (DPT) against diphtheria, whooping cough and tetanus at the third, fourth and fifth months of life; polio oral vaccine also at the third, fourth and fifth months; measles vaccine at the sixth, seventh and eighth months; and smallpox vaccination at the ninth month of life.

Can this immunization schedule be changed without adversely affecting the child?

Yes. It is often varied at the doctor's discretion.

What are so-called "booster shots"?

These are additional injections given a year or two after the original immunization in order to maintain immunity.

When are the booster injections given?

For diphtheria, whooping cough, and tetanus, at about eighteen months of age; then every two years thereafter until school age; then every three years until puberty.

Polio booster injections should be given seven months after the first two injections, and possibly one more injection should be given a year later.

Is the effectiveness of these injections lost if the interval is prolonged because of an illness the child may have?

In general, no. The intervals may be prolonged for several weeks or even months without affecting the value of immunizations.

Should inoculations against disease be given if the child is sick from another cause?

No. Injections should be postponed when the child has a cold or other illness.

What are the reactions to injections against these contagious diseases?

Usually there are none, or they are very mild. Occasionally, one notices irritability, fever, restlessness, lack of appetite, or vomiting. These symptoms do not last for more than a day or two.

Are there any local reactions in the area that injections are given?

In some cases, there is redness and swelling in the area, but this usually passes within a day or two.

Is it common for a small lump to appear at the site where an injection was given?

Yes, but this has no significance and will disappear within a few days.

What is the treatment for reactions to immunization in children?

A small dose of aspirin as prescribed by your doctor. Also, do not bathe the child for a day or two.

On what part of the body are injections usually given?

In the buttock or in the outer part of the upper arm.

Who usually gives immunization injections?

Your physician or his regular nurse-assistant.

If there is a marked reaction to an injection, is it wise to inform your physician?

Yes. This information may influence him to reduce the dose of the next injection or to spread the series of injections over four to five injections instead of the usual two or three.

Is it ever necessary to discontinue immunization injections entirely?

If the child is highly allergic to egg, it may be wise not to give measles vaccine.

Are there ever any harmful effects from immunization injections?

Just one or two patients among millions may have a serious reaction. The beneficial effects far outweigh any possible harm that may come from immunization injections.

Can allergic people be given immunization injections?

Yes, though it may be wise to give the diphtheria, whooping cough, and tetanus immunizations separately. Also, smaller amounts may have to be given at each injection.

THE SCHICK TEST

What is the Schick test?

This is a test to determine whether a child is immune or has developed an immunity (by injections) to diphtheria.

How is the Schick test done?

A small amount of toxin is injected into the skin of the forearm and the reaction is noted two to four days later. If nothing appears on the arm, the test is called negative, and the child is judged to be immune to diphtheria.

What is a positive Schick test?

If there is an area of redness and thickening of the skin the size of a dime, it is called a positive Schick test and shows that the child is not immune.

Does the Schick test cause the child to become sick in any way?

No.

How often are Schick tests done?

Some physicians recommend doing them every year; others feel that the tests are not necessary, since booster injections of the diphtheria vaccine will insure immunity.

What should be done if there is a positive Schick test?

The child should be given the complete course of injections against diphtheria.

SMALLPOX VACCINATION

How is smallpox vaccination given?

This is done by the scratch or multiple puncture method.

Does smallpox vaccine ever produce the disease?

No.

Where is smallpox vaccine best given?

It is best to vaccinate on the outer surface of the upper arm, usually the left arm, near the shoulder.

Can people be vaccinated on the thigh?

Yes, but there is more danger of contamination by stool or urine in that area.

Is there any immediate reaction to smallpox vaccination?

No.

When does the positive reaction to smallpox vaccination set in?

In four to five days, a red spot will appear and become larger and will form a blister. At about the eighth to ninth day, the blister is quite large and is surrounded by an area of redness the size of a quarter or a half-dollar. Thereafter, the blister dries up, leaving a crust, and the redness begins to subside and disappear within about two weeks after the original vaccination.

Is smallpox vaccination accompanied by fever and other signs of illness?

Yes, during the second week, when the vaccination reacts and is at its height. Temperatures as high as 103° to 104° may be recorded during this period.

What is the treatment for the vaccination reaction?

It is wise to give aspirin in doses recommended by your doctor. Cool sponges to the body may be given if the temperature is high.

Are there any other signs of severe vaccination reaction?

Yes. There may be swelling in the armpit near the site of the vaccination. This does not necessarily indicate that an infection has set in.

If the vaccination seems to be exceptionally red, swollen, and painful, should the patient see his doctor?

Yes.

Does the patient ever develop a rash from smallpox vaccination?

In a small percentage of cases, a mild rash may appear. This will disappear as the reaction subsides.

Is it necessary to keep a dressing on the vaccination?

No. In fact, it is preferable not to have a dressing.

Should a vaccination shield be used?

Definitely not.

Should the vaccination area be bathed?

No. It is preferable to keep the area dry until the inflammation has subsided completely and a firm crust has formed.

Can a child be bathed and the arm wet when the scab on a vaccination is dry?

Yes.

Does one ever encounter secondary vaccinations?

Yes. Sometimes there may be a small blister near the original large vaccination. This will cause no harm.

How long does it usually take for the scab to fall off?

Between two and three weeks. It is best to allow it to fall off by itself.

Does it do any harm if the vaccination scab is rubbed off accidentally?

No.

Does the vaccination usually leave a large scar?

Nowadays the scar is usually quite small.

What should be done if the smallpox vaccination does not "take"?

It should be done over again, after a wait of two to four weeks from the original vaccination.

Is it necessary to continue vaccinations until there is a positive "take"?

Yes.

Should a baby be vaccinated when he has a cold?

No.

Should a baby with eczema be vaccinated?

No. Even if the child has had a rash or a skin condition for a period of months or years, the vaccination should be delayed. *Never* vaccinate a child while he has a rash!

Should a baby be vaccinated if another child in the family has eczema?

No. It is easy for the virus to be transmitted from the baby to the other child, with possible serious consequences.

Do vaccinations often become infected?

No. This is a common misconception.

615

How often should a child be revaccinated?

Every five to seven years.

Does a child need to be revaccinated when entering school?

No.

Are there ever any convulsions from vaccination?

Rarely. They are caused by the high fever accompanying some vaccinations.

What are the chances of encephalitis (inflammation of the brain) from smallpox vaccination?

This is extremely rare, occurring perhaps once in five hundred thousand vaccinations.

Does this encephalitis occur in young infants?

Not usually. It occurs more often in children who are vaccinated for the first time after they are five years of age. This is the main reason pediatricians prefer to vaccinate children early.

Do adults ever get encephalitis as a result of smallpox vaccination?

No.

Can the encephalitis which occurs from vaccination be successfully treated?

Yes. It should also be remembered that the dangers of getting smallpox from not being vaccinated are much greater than the dangers of getting encephalitis from smallpox vaccination.

Will schools permit children to enter who have not been vaccinated?

No. Practically every community in the United States requires a vaccination certificate.

How effective is smallpox vaccination?

If there has been a positive "take," it will protect completely against this disease.

POLIOMYELITIS VACCINATION

Should polio vaccination be given if a patient is ill?

No. It is best to wait until he has recovered from any illness.

Is polio vaccine safe?

Yes. It is completely safe.

Can polio vaccine produce poliomyelitis?

No! Early difficulties in manufacture have been overcome completely and it is now perfectly safe to give both the oral and the Salk types of vaccine.

How effective is polio vaccination?

It is considered to be tremendously effective and will prevent the disease in more than 85 to 90 per cent of those vaccinated. Those who may get it despite vaccination will get a very mild form of the disease, often without paralysis.

Can allergic people be given polio vaccine?

Yes. There have been no serious effects in allergic patients.

Are there usually reactions to polio vaccination?

No. Occasionally, there may be very slight fever or irritability for a day.

Are any special precautions necessary after polio vaccination?

No.

Does the polio vaccine contain penicillin?

The Salk type for injection does contain a small amount. The oral Sabin vaccine does not.

Can people who are sensitive to penicillin be given polio injections?

Yes. There have been no serious reactions even in people sensitive to penicillin.

617

Is it permissible to give polio vaccine at the same time as other vaccines?

Yes.

Is it permissible to vaccinate against polio at any time of the year?

Yes.

How soon after a full course of oral polio vaccine does immunity develop?

Within a period of several weeks.

Is it necessary, after the three oral doses of polio vaccine, to repeat the course within the next year or two?

No. It is thought that the full course of oral vaccine will produce a permanent immunity. However, just to be safe, some pediatricians do prescribe a second course of vaccine a few years after the original one.

Should older children and adults be given the polio vaccine?

Yes. Only in this way can the disease be totally and permanently eradicated as an epidemic menace.

If a person has already had polio, will he benefit from vaccination?

Yes. The vaccine will increase his immunity. Also, he may have immunity to only one strain of the polio virus; the vaccine will give him immunity to other strains as well.

Should polio vaccination be withheld if the child is going to have his tonsils removed?

No.

Is there any way to tell if someone is immune to polio before the vaccine is given?

Yes, but the procedure is not practical for everyday use. It is a very expensive test and takes a long time to perform. Also, there are only a few laboratories in the country equipped to perform such a test.

MEASLES VACCINATION

Is there a satisfactory method of immunizing against measles?

Yes. The new measles vaccine is about 90 per cent effective.

At what age should measles vaccination be carried out?

When the child is about 6 months old.

How is measles vaccination done?

There are two methods at present; by giving either the killed measles virus or the weakened live virus.

What are the two different methods of vaccination?

1. The killed measles vaccine is given by injection preferably at monthly intervals for three injections starting when the child is 6 months of age.
2. The live virus vaccine is given all at one time along with an injection of gamma globulin.

Are the two methods of measles vaccination equally effective?

Yes.

Do the reactions to the two types of measles vaccination differ?

Yes. The temperature reaction and feeling of illness is somewhat less when the killed virus three-injection method is used. However, improvement in the live virus vaccine has reduced reactions markedly.

What is the reaction to measles vaccination among children?

In about one out of four or five cases, a fever, upper respiratory congestion, and a slight rash appears within a few days after vaccination. Recovery is prompt within two to three days.

Are there any children who should not be given the measles vaccine?

Yes. Those who are allergic to egg may develop a severe reaction.

619

SCARLET FEVER IMMUNIZATION

Are there any immunizing injections against scarlet fever?

Yes, but they are not given any more. The antibiotic drugs are so effective in the treatment of this disease that immunization is unnecessary.

TYPHOID FEVER VACCINATION

When is typhoid fever immunization given?

When the child or adult is going into an area where there is danger of exposure to typhoid fever. This applies particularly to certain foreign countries.

What is the routine immunization against typhoid fever?

A series of three injections into the skin or beneath the skin, given one to two weeks apart.

What vaccine is used?

Usually a vaccine containing the dead typhoid and paratyphoid germs.

Are injections against typhoid fever effective?

Yes.

Are there any reactions to typhoid immunization?

Yes. The arm may become very red and swollen and there may be fever for a few days.

What is the best treatment for the reaction to typhoid immunization?

Aspirin and bed rest.

Are booster injections necessary after typhoid immunization?

Yes. One injection a year of a small dose of the vaccine should be given if a patient is again going to an area where there is danger of contracting typhoid.

OTHER IMMUNIZATIONS

Are there any effective immunizations against the common cold?

No, although many so-called "cold shots" are in use today.

Is there any vaccine against mumps?

Yes, but it is not used routinely because it is only moderately effective and the immunity is not long-lasting.

Is there any immunization against tuberculosis?

Yes, there is a vaccine called BCG. (See Chapter 68, on Tuberculosis.)

Is vaccination against tuberculosis effective?

There is great controversy on this subject; the vaccine is not generally used in this country.

When is tuberculosis vaccination advised?

In certain situations, when the individual has been exposed for long periods of time to a known case of tuberculosis, it will be advised.

Is there an effective immunization against rabies?

Yes.

When is vaccination against rabies given?

When an individual has been bitten by any animal that is suspected of being rabid, such as a dog, cat, fox, squirrel, rabbit, rat, wolf, etc.

Are rabies immunization injections given in every case of dog bite?

No. They are given when the dog is known or suspected of being diseased. The dog must be sent to a place where he can be held and examined for a few days to note whether he develops rabies. If the dog is found to be healthy, no immunization is necessary.

If the animal that has caused the bite cannot be found, should the injections be given?

Yes, as a safeguard.

How is rabies inoculation carried out?

By daily injections for fourteen days.

Is there any effective treatment for rabies once it has developed?

No. There is a very high mortality rate once a child or adult has developed the disease.

What is the best local treatment for a dog bite?

Thorough washing of the area with soap and water for at least ten to twenty minutes.

Should a dog-bite wound be cauterized?

No. This treatment was given up years ago because it does not safeguard against rabies if the animal was afflicted with the disease.

If the skin has not been broken by a dog bite is there any danger of infection?

Not usually, but the area should still be washed thoroughly with soap and water for ten to twenty minutes.

Should a dog bite be reported to the authorities?

Yes. In almost all communities it is the law that such bites be reported to the police or to the Board of Health.

Does it make any difference where the animal has bitten the patient?

Yes. The closer to the head the bite is, the more serious it is.

Are there any dangers from giving rabies inoculations?

No, but it is a painful process to have to endure.

Are there any effective vaccinations against typhus fever, cholera, yellow fever, and the plague?

Yes. There are very effective vaccinations against all of these diseases.

When should vaccinations against typhus fever, cholera, yellow fever, or the plague be given?

Only when one is traveling to an area where there is danger of contracting these diseases.

What immunization procedures are necessary for travel to foreign countries?

a. Smallpox. This is required for re-entry into the United States and is also required for entry into some foreign countries. The traveler must be vaccinated against smallpox within three years of the date of travel; a certificate of such vaccination is required by law.

b. Typhoid and paratyphoid fever. Vaccinations against these diseases are advisable in travel to countries where these diseases are prevalent.

c. Tetanus. It is advisable to be injected against tetanus if there is a danger of injury during one's travel. However, this is not required by law.

Where can one get additional information on immunizations necessary for foreign travel?

The United States Department of Health, Education and Welfare, and the Public Health Service issue a booklet giving exact details of immunization procedures advisable for travelers. The World Health Organization issues a standard certificate that can be filled in by your physician. It lists the injections and the dates on which they have been given.

623

Disease	Material Used	When Given	Number of Injections	Spacing Injectio
MUMPS	Mumps vaccine	During adolescence or adulthood	2	1 week
CHICKENPOX	None	. . .		. . .
INFECTIOUS HEPATITIS	Gamma globulin	Exposure to case of infectious hepatitis	1	. . .
SCARLET FEVER	Penicillin	Exposure to case of scarlet fever	3	Daily
RABIES	Rabies vaccine	Following suspicious animal bite	14	Daily
CHOLERA	Cholera vaccine	°For foreign travel	2–3	1 week
TYPHUS FEVER	Typhus vaccine	°For foreign travel	2–3	1 week
YELLOW FEVER	Yellow fever vaccine	°For foreign travel	1	. . .
PLAGUE	Plague vaccine	°For foreign travel	2–3	1 week
INFLUENZA	Influenza vaccine	During epidemics	2	1 week
ROCKY MOUNTAIN SPOTTED FEVER	Rocky Mountain spotted fever vaccine	For persons exposed to tick in suspicious areas	3	1 week

° *Needed only in traveling to countries where these diseases are present—as in Asia, Africa, and some parts of Europe, Central and South America.*

actions	Duration of Immunity	"Recall" or Booster Injections	Remarks
t to be giv- egg-sensi- eople	Unknown	. . .	Not used in children before adolescence
. .	. . .	. . .	. . .
None	4–6 weeks	None	. . .
None	4–6 weeks	Same procedure if re-exposed	May give penicillin only in adequate dosage
Slight	3–6 months	If bitten again after 3 months	May not need full series if dog is found not infected
Slight	Short	Every 6–12 months	. . .
Slight	Short	Every 12 months	. . .
y be mod- erate	Long	Every 6 years	. . .
Slight	Short	Every 6–12 months	. . .
Slight	Short		. . .
Moderate	Short	Annually	. . .

ust be careful of reactions in allergic people sensitive to eggs.

Disease	Material Used	When Given	Number of Injections	Spacing Injectio
DIPHTHERIA	Diphtheria fluid toxoid	Infancy and childhood, or up- on exposure	3	1 month
WHOOPING COUGH	Pertussis vaccine	Infancy and childhood, or up- on exposure	3	1 month
TETANUS	Tetanus fluid toxoid	Infancy and childhood, or af- ter injury	3	1 month
SMALLPOX	Cowpox virus	Infancy, child- hood, and adult- hood	1	. . .
POLIOMYELITIS	Salk polio vac- cine	Infancy — to age 40 years, or older	3–4	First two tions 1 m apart, thir jection 7 m later
	Sabin polio vaccine	3, 4, 5 months of age	No injections. 3 oral doses	1 month ap
TYPHOID FEVER	Typhoid, paraty- phoid vaccine	At any age when traveling to sus- picious area	3	1–4 wee
MEASLES	Gamma globulin	On exposure to case of measles	1	. . .
	Killed or live measles virus	At 6, 7, or 8 months of age	3 of killed— 1 of live virus	1 month ap
GERMAN MEASLES	Gamma globulin	Exposure to Ger- man measles	1	. . .

ACCINATION CHART

actions	Duration of Immunity	"Recall" or Booster Injections	Remarks
e to slight	Varies		
t to mod-erate	Varies	1st booster—after 1 year 2nd and 3rd—2 year intervals 4th and 5th—3 year intervals and on exposure to disease	All three (diphtheria, tetanus and whooping cough) may be combined in a single injection — in young children only
e to slight	Varies		
Ioderate	Several years	5–7 years, and for foreign travel	. . .
None	Unknown—probably long	4th injection, one year after third injection	. . .
None	Probably permanent	Not necessary	The best protection is obtained by administration of both types of vaccine
ioderate	1–3 years	Every 1–3 years	. . .
None	4–6 weeks	. . .	Best to give modifying dose so child will develop modified measles
Ioderate	Unknown	Yearly	. . .
None	4–6 weeks	. . .	Only given if patient is pregnant, during first 3 months

IMMUNIZATION CHART

PRESENT ACCEPTED IDEAL SCHEDULE FOR INFANTS AND CHILDREN

Age

Age	
3 months	1st diphtheria, whooping cough, tetanus (DPT) (combined in 1 injection). 1st dose of oral polio vaccine.
4 months	2nd diphtheria, whooping cough, tetanus (DPT) injection. 2nd dose of oral polio vaccine.
5 months	3rd diphtheria, whooping cough, tetanus (DPT) injection. 3rd dose of oral polio vaccine.
6 months	1st measles vaccine injection.
7 months	2nd measles vaccine injection.
8 months	3rd measles vaccine injection.
9 months	Smallpox vaccination.
18 months	Booster diphtheria, whooping cough, tetanus injection.
18 months	Possible booster dose of oral polio vaccine.
20 months	Possible booster measles vaccine injection.
3½ years	Booster diphtheria, whooping cough, tetanus.
6 years	Booster diphtheria, whooping cough, tetanus.
9 years	Booster diphtheria and tetanus (combined).
12 years	Booster tetanus.

Additional boosters:

Measles—additional dose 1 year after original course.

Pertussis—after exposure to a case of pertussis.

Diphtheria—after exposure to a case of diphtheria.

Tetanus—after injury from rusty object or one contaminated by dirt. Such additional boosters may be advisable for any suspicious injury causing a puncture wound.

Smallpox vaccination—every 5 to 7 years, or if there is any suspicious case in the community. Also, before traveling to a foreign country, if not previously vaccinated in preceding three years.

Polio—fourth injection one year after third injection.

29 *Infant and*

Childhood Diseases

(See Chapter 16, on Child Behavior; Chapter 17, on Contagious
Diseases; Chapter 30, on Infant Feeding; Chapter 43,
on the Newborn Child.)

C R O U P

What is croup (catarrhal laryngitis)?

It is an inflammatory disease of the respiratory passage, involving
the larynx or voice box and occurring mostly in children between
the ages of one and five.

What causes croup?

It is caused by a virus infection in most cases. Bacterial organisms
also may be the causative agent.

Does diphtheria cause croup?

Yes. There is a type of diphtheritic croup in which a membrane is
formed in the larynx and trachea.

How can croup be recognized?

The first symptoms are difficulty in breathing, hoarseness or loss of
voice, coughing, crowing, and a barking sound similar to that made
by a seal. There is a slight elevation of temperature in the average
case, but it may be considerably elevated in the severe case.

629

When does croup usually start?

At night. It tends to subside during the day and then to become worse again the next night.

How long does the average case of croup last?

About one to three days.

What is the treatment for croup?

a. Steam inhalations. Care must be exercised not to burn the child.

b. Make the child vomit by putting a spoon down to the back of his throat. Vomiting often causes the child to expel an obstructing plug of mucus from the throat.

c. Give ipecac, under a doctor's supervision, to induce vomiting.

d. Keep the room warm and moist by having a steam kettle going.

Steam Inhalation for Croup. The old-fashioned croup kettle is still effective but has been replaced by an apparatus of the type shown below, which can be purchased at almost any drugstore. Electric steam inhalators benefit children with croup by moistening and warming the air.

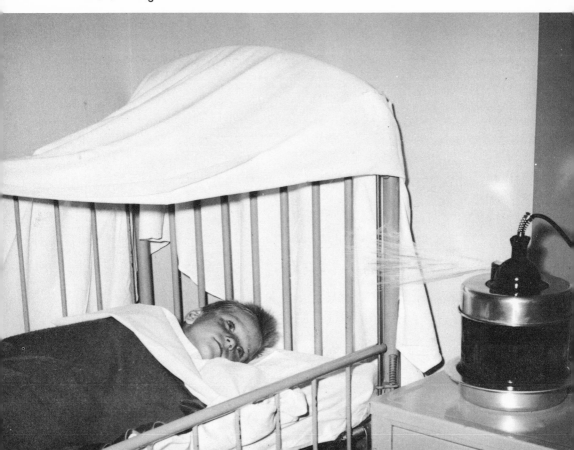

Does croup tend to recur?

Yes. Children who have once had an attack of croup tend to have repeated attacks with each respiratory infection during the next two to three years.

Do the severe forms of croup require special treatment?

Yes. It is imperative that children with severe croup be seen by a doctor immediately, because in the severe case there is a great tendency toward obstruction of breathing.

What should be done in severe cases of croup?

Where there is obstruction to the breathing which is not relieved by steam, it may be necessary for the doctor to admit the child to the hospital for an immediate tracheotomy. In dire emergencies, the physician may carry out this procedure in the home.

What is a tracheotomy?

It is an opening made into the windpipe to allow the child to breathe.

Is there any other treatment for severe croup?

Yes. Many cases will be benefited by giving oxygen.

Are antibiotics effective against croup?

They are usually not necessary in the mild form, but they are helpful in the severe cases.

What special diet should be given to children with croup?

It is preferable to give only warm fluids and soft foods.

Is there any way to prevent croup?

No, except to provide good humidity in the home, particularly in the room in which the child sleeps.

Is there any effective vaccine against croup?

No.

Are there permanent after-effects of croup?

Usually not. The great majority of cases make a complete recovery.

Is it necessary to quarantine a child with croup?

No, but the disease is somewhat contagious and the same precautions should be taken as for any ordinary upper respiratory infection.

Does croup tend to occur more often in allergic children?

Yes.

Does it occur more often during one particular season?

Yes. It occurs more frequently in the winter and fall months.

When may the child be allowed out of doors after recovery from croup?

In mild cases, after two to three days; in severe cases, after a week to ten days.

CELIAC DISEASE

What is celiac disease?

It is a disturbance of the digestive system, chiefly involving the digestion of starches and fats.

What causes this disease?

A failure or deficiency of some of the enzymes involved in the digestive process. There is also a disturbance in absorption of fats.

How often does celiac disease occur?

About one in a hundred children has this condition.

Does it tend to run in families?

Yes.

Is there any relationship to allergies?

Yes. We seem to find more of these cases in families that have a history of allergies. Some of the children with this condition later manifest allergic symptoms as well.

When does celiac disease become evident?

Usually during the first year of life. The baby may appear to be normal at first, and then begin to show signs of this condition between six and eighteen months of age.

How does this condition manifest itself?

By alternate periods of diarrhea and constipation, with large, bulky, foul-smelling stools. The infant fails to gain weight, and may even lose weight. The abdomen becomes large and distended, the buttocks become small and flabby. The appetite is poor, and occasionally there may be some vomiting. Also, the infant is subject to frequent colds and bronchitis, and may have a chronic cough.

Are there varying degrees of severity of celiac disease?

Yes. There are very mild cases which are difficult to diagnose, and severe forms which can be easily recognized.

What tests can be done to make a positive diagnosis?

The stool is examined for the presence of undigested fats and starches, and also for the presence of trypsin, one of the digestive enzymes.

There are also certain tests to determine the absorption of vitamin A, gelatin, and glucose into the blood from the stomach and duodenum.

Will x-rays help in the diagnosis of this condition?

Yes, sometimes gastro-intestinal studies will help in the diagnosis.

What is the treatment for celiac disease?

The child must be kept on a special diet for a long time, usually with antibiotics added to control infections. The diet will be high in proteins, low in fat, with no starches or sugars (other than natural fruit sugar).

What milk is used?

A special high-protein, low-fat milk is usually used, and continued for many months.

What solids are tolerated by the child with celiac disease?

Bananas, raw fruits, and fat-free meats are usually well tolerated. Some vegetables can be taken. Pot cheese or fat-free cottage cheese will usually not cause difficulty.

Can the baby have the usual vitamins?

The water-soluble multivitamin preparations are given, usually in increased amounts because of the difficulty in absorption.

What further changes are made?

As the infant tolerates the above foods and stools improve, other foods are added gradually. The last foods given are starches, cereals, butter and cream, and whole milk.

How long does the infant stay on this diet?

About six months to two years.

Is recovery usually complete in celiac disease?

Yes.

Can the child take a full diet later in life?

Yes.

Are there any setbacks during the treatment?

Yes. Any infection, teething, or addition of a restricted food may cause a setback. Sometimes even without any change there may be a temporary setback.

How does this diet affect the child's disposition?

Some children take the diet well, eat avidly, and may take large amounts of the special milk and bananas without any disturbance.

Others seem to get bored by the diet, so the mother must use her ingenuity to get the child to eat the foods prescribed.

Can celiac disease be treated satisfactorily at home?

Yes. Hospitalization may be necessary only in the beginning of the disease or for thorough investigation and diagnosis.

Does the baby have to stay in bed with this condition?

No, except during an acute illness.

Will celiac disease clear up without treatment?

No. If the baby stays on a full diet the stools become worse, weight loss increases, and severe infections are more apt to occur.

Does celiac disease tend to recur?

In some cases it may be necessary to continue modified dietary care for several years. Otherwise there may be relapses or recurrences, especially when infections occur.

How often are changes in diet made?

Usually, it is best to have the physician check the infant every month, to make diet changes and observe his progress. Later on, the child should be checked every two to three months until recovery is complete.

Is the pancreas involved in this condition?

Probably not, though doctors are not sure. It may be mildly affected.

Is pancreatic extract used in treatment?

In some cases, it will give beneficial results; in others, it will have no added value.

PANCREATIC CYSTIC FIBROSIS

What is pancreatic cystic fibrosis?

It is a disease somewhat similar in its manifestations to celiac disease, but it is more severe in nature and tends to have more complications, such as lung infections.

How often does it occur?

About one in five hundred to six hundred babies has this disease.

When does it start?

It starts earlier than celiac disease, usually from birth to six months of age.

Does it tend to run in families?

Yes.

Does heat affect these children inordinately?

Yes. They lose a great deal of salt in the sweat secretions and may go into collapse on a hot summer's day.

Do some children die with pancreatic cystic fibrosis?

Yes. Some cases may die during a heat spell, others may die of pulmonary complications, and still others from malnutrition. About 50 per cent die before the age of five.

What is the treatment for pancreatic cystic fibrosis?

Diet similar to that in celiac disease, adequate salt intake, large amounts of vitamins, constant use of antibiotics to prevent infections, and the giving of pancreatic extracts.

How long does treatment have to be continued to maintain these children?

For several years, after which time the condition usually disappears.

Is this disease caused by disturbed pancreatic function?

Yes. There is involvement of the pancreas, with cyst formation. This leads to insufficiency of pancreatic enzymes which are necessary for the digestion of starches and fats.

Are any other organs involved in this disease?

Yes. Excessive mucous production and excessive viscosity (thick-

636

ness) of that mucus may also be present in the lungs and in areas of the intestinal tract.

If there is a case of this disease in the family should the parents plan to have other children?

Yes. They may have additional children, but they should be told that there is a one in four chance that another child will have the same condition.

Are there any special tests for this disease?

The same tests as are used in making the diagnosis of celiac disease. In addition, some recent tests have been devised to test the salt content of the sweat.

Is it easy to differentiate this condition from celiac disease?

In very frank cases, the two can be differentiated, but in mild ones it may be difficult to tell them apart.

HIRSCHSPRUNG'S DISEASE
(Megacolon)

(See Chapter 61, on the Small and Large Intestine.)

What is Hirschsprung's disease?

It is a disease, present from birth, involving the large intestine, in which there is a contracted segment in the sigmoid colon on the left side, with tremendous dilatation and enlargement of the remainder of the bowel above the constricted portion.

How common is Hirschsprung's disease?

It is a relatively rare condition, seen more often among males, and constitutes about one of every ten thousand hospital admissions.

What causes Hirschsprung's disease?

It is thought to be due to a developmental deformity in which certain nerves are lacking in the contracted portion of the bowel (sigmoid colon). This lack prevents the involved segment of bowel from relaxing and dilating. In order to propel the feces forward, the bowel above the constriction enlarges, and because it is difficult to get gas and feces beyond the contracted area, the bowel above dilates tremendously.

How is the diagnosis of Hirschsprung's disease made?

By characteristic findings on x-ray examination with the giving of barium to outline the bowel.

What is the course and treatment of this condition?

Mild cases tend to improve and get well with medical management over a period of years. The majority of severe cases will require the surgical removal of the constricted portion of large intestine.

Is surgery successful in curing Hirschsprung's disease?

Yes. Modern techniques have improved greatly and the surgical treatment of this condition is now safe and can promise an extremely high rate of cure.

NEPHROSIS

(See Chapter 33, on the Kidney and the Ureter.)

RHEUMATIC FEVER

(See Chapter 57, on Rheumatic Fever.)

ERYTHROBLASTOSIS

What is erythroblastosis?

A disease of the newborn due to an incompatibility between the mother's blood and the newborn infant's blood.

What are other names for this disease?

a. Rh factor disease.
b. Severe jaundice of the newborn.
c. Severe anemia of the newborn.

What is meant by the "Rh factor"?

All people are either Rh positive or Rh negative. This means that the blood contains a substance (Rh substance) in Rh positive people which is not present in Rh negative people.

What percentage of people are Rh positive?

Eighty-five per cent. The other 15 per cent are Rh negative.

Are these blood factors transmitted from parent to child?

Yes.

In what type of marriages may we get the Rh factor disease?

Only when the woman is Rh negative and the man Rh positive.

Will all the babies of such a marriage develop this disease?

No. Only about one in two hundred babies born of such a marriage will have this condition.

What brings about this condition?

An Rh negative mother carries an Rh positive baby in her uterus. Some of the Rh positive baby blood substance gets into the mother's circulation and produces Rh positive antibodies. These antibodies in turn will later get into the baby's circulation and destroy the baby's own blood cells.

How does this affect the newborn infant?

By producing anemia due to destruction of the infant's red blood cells, thus producing jaundice (yellow skin and eyes).

How is the jaundice produced?

The infant's liver is unable to clear all the destroyed cells from the circulation, causing an overflow of bile into the circulation.

How can this condition be recognized?

The infant becomes pale and jaundiced during the first twenty-four hours of life. In addition, the liver and spleen are found to be enlarged. Blood tests will show the presence of the antibodies in the infant's blood.

How does the jaundice in the Rh factor disease differ from normal newborn jaundice?

By its very early development, in the first twenty-four hours, and its severity.

Is there any way to determine during the pregnancy whether the baby may have this disease?

Yes. Every mother should be tested in advance to determine whether she is Rh positive or Rh negative. If she is Rh negative, her blood should be tested frequently during the latter weeks and months of her pregnancy for the presence and amount of these specific antibodies. If they are present, the baby may develop this disease.

What is the treatment for erythroblastosis?

As soon after birth as possible an exchange transfusion should be done.

What is meant by an "exchange transfusion"?

An attempt is made to remove all, or nearly all, of the baby's blood and replace it with blood from a donor—blood that does not contain these dangerous antibodies. This procedure will require the services of an expert in the field.

Is it ever necessary to give more than one exchange transfusion?

Yes. In some cases the jaundice may reappear in two to three days, necessitating a second, and in rare cases, even a third exchange transfusion.

Can exchange transfusion cure erythroblastosis?

Yes. If done early enough, it will cure almost every case.

What can happen in an untreated case of erythroblastosis?

The baby may die in a few days because of the extreme blood destruction, or the intense jaundice may permanently injure certain parts of the brain.

What is the nature of this brain injury?

It may produce spasticity or extreme drowsiness in the baby, and may later be the cause of mental retardation, convulsions, and a form of cerebral palsy.

Can exchange transfusion prevent brain injury?

Yes. By removing the antibodies and the jaundice-producing substance it will prevent brain injury. It must be done very early, however, and may need to be repeated if jaundice recurs.

Does Rh factor disease ever produce stillbirths before the baby is delivered?

Yes. In some cases it is a cause of death in the uterus or just before birth. In some Rh negative women we may get a history of repeated stillbirths due to this disease.

Is it possible to have a live baby in such cases?

Yes. If the condition is recognized during pregnancy, the live infant may be taken prematurely by Cesarean section or by prompting premature labor. An exchange transfusion is done immediately after birth.

Are first-born babies ever affected with erythroblastosis?

Not ordinarily. It usually affects later pregnancies. It may affect a first-born infant if the mother has been given a transfusion or blood injection with Rh positive blood some time prior to her first pregnancy. Then, her blood may contain the dangerous antibodies as a result of the previous blood injection.

Is there any other mechanism that can produce erythroblastosis besides the Rh factor?

Yes. In a small number of cases of so-called ABO incompatibility, in which the mother's blood group is "O" and the baby's group is "A" or "B," a mild form of this disease may be produced.

What proportion of cases are caused by ABO incompatibility?

About 5 to 10 per cent.

How long does the baby have to stay in the hospital after an exchange transfusion?

For about a week, to make sure that there is no recurrence of anemia or jaundice.

Does he require any other special treatments?

No.

May a child who has recovered from erythroblastosis be breast-fed?

Yes. There was a time when the possible introduction of these antibodies (some of which may be present in the breast milk) into the baby's stomach was feared. It is now known that they cause no harm when introduced in that manner.

Does the baby need any special care after he leaves the hospital?

Yes. It is wise to keep checking his blood every two weeks for about two months, and then every month for several months thereafter. Usually, no further treatment is necessary.

Is there any way to prevent the development of these antibodies in the mother during subsequent pregnancies?

No. Several methods have been tried, including the use of cortisone, but they have not been successful.

AMAUROTIC FAMILY IDIOCY
(Tay-Sachs disease)

What is amaurotic family idiocy?

It is a fatal disease of young infants associated with blindness and mental retardation.

What are the manifestations of this disease?

A baby will progress normally until about six months of age, then he will stop in his development and regress. He will show signs of blindness, apathy, weakness of his muscles, and later spasticity and convulsions.

What causes this condition?

The infant is unable to utilize certain fatty substances in his food. These substances then accumulate in the brain, causing destruction of the normal brain cells.

How is the diagnosis of this condition made?

By examination of the eyes with an ophthalmoscope. A characteristic abnormal "cherry-red spot" will be seen on the retina.

Does this disease run in families?

Yes. If a family has one baby with this condition there is a one in four chance that another baby born to these parents will have the same condition.

Does amaurotic family idiocy occur only in Jewish families?

Almost exclusively. About 95 per cent of the cases occur in Jewish families.

Is there any treatment for this condition?

None.

Is there any way of preventing this disease?

No.

Is it always fatal?

Yes.

How long can a baby live with this condition?

About two to three years. The baby's nutrition goes steadily downhill, there is loss of weight and increasing spasticity, until the baby eventually dies.

Is it necessary to put a child with this condition in a hospital?

No, as there is little that can be done in a hospital that cannot be done at home. However, in certain instances it may be wiser to place the baby in a chronic-disease hospital or institution so as not to excessively encumber the home environment. The presence of such a baby in a home may have a bad psychological effect upon the parents and other children.

NIEMANN-PICK DISEASE

What is Niemann-Pick Disease?

It is similar to Tay-Sachs disease, with the added element of a large spleen and liver. It, too, involves blindness, the cherry-red spot in the eye, and the mental retardation.

Is this also familial, and does it tend to occur in Jewish families?

Yes.

Is this also fatal before three years of age?

Yes.

MONGOLISM

What is Mongolism?

It is a form of mental retardation occurring in three of every thousand newborns.

How is Mongolism recognized?

By the appearance of the child. His head is usually small, the muscles are flabby, the face has a characteristic appearance: eyes slanting upward and outward, a wide nasal bridge, and a protruding tongue. The hand is broad and spadelike, the palmar creases are not normal, the neck is short and broad, and there may be an abnormal heart condition present.

What causes Mongolism?

The cause is unknown. It is possibly due to a defect in development during the early part of a pregnancy.

Is Mongolism hereditary?

No.

Does it occur more often with older mothers than young ones?

Yes.

Does it occur more often after several normal babies than as a first baby?

Yes.

Is there any special blood or x-ray test to be sure of the diagnosis?

No. Certain skull x-rays may give a clue to the condition.

Is there any treatment for Mongolism?

No.

Is there any way of preventing it?

No.

Do these children grow up?

Yes; they can live many years. There are Mongolism cases that have lived to forty years of age.

What is the level of intelligence that Mongolism cases can reach?

They usually remain infantile or childlike all their lives.

What is the usual disposition of children with Mongolism?

They are usually pleasant, affectionate, almost doll-like at times. They are rarely disobedient, have no aggressiveness, temper tantrums, or behavior difficulties.

Can they be cared for in the home?

Yes. In many cases they can stay at home. However, if there are other children in the family who would be adversely affected psychologically by the presence of a Mongolism case in the home, then perhaps it may be advisable to admit the child to an institution.

What institutions will take care of Mongolism cases?

Any institution that will take mentally retarded children. In most states there is a special hospital that will care for them.

Can children with Mongolism be educated?

To a limited degree.

Can they be taught a trade?

Yes. They can be taught simple tasks and simple occupations.

Can they be made self-supporting?

Rarely, though occasionally a case of "high-grade Mongolism" can be taught an occupation, such as errand boy, and can become self-supporting.

Why is this condition called Mongolism?

Because of the facial appearance and the upward slant of the eyes.

Does Mongolism occur only in the white race?

No. It occurs in all races.

RETROLENTAL FIBROPLASIA

What is retrolental fibroplasia?

This is a form of blindness that used to occur in very small premature babies and in some children who were born by Cesarean section.

What causes this disease?

Until recently, the cause was unknown. It has now been ascertained that retrolental fibroplasia was caused by *oxygen poisoning!*

Oxygen is a beneficial, lifesaving gas; how can there be "oxygen poisoning"?

Too much oxygen, when given to very small premature babies, interferes with normal eye development and can lead to blindness in some cases.

How much oxygen is used now for premature babies?

No more than 40 per cent of the air they breathe in an incubator.

Do all premature babies require extra oxygen?

No; only those who appear to have difficulty in breathing.

Can retrolental fibroplasia be cured?

The very early cases may be helped, but the later cases cannot.

HYALINE MEMBRANE DISEASE

What is hyaline membrane disease?

It is a disease of premature babies, and some Cesarean babies, in which there is an interference with the normal breathing mechanism.

When does it develop?

Usually within six to twenty-four hours after birth.

Are babies born with hyaline membrane disease?

It is difficult to tell at birth. These infants seem normal at birth and for several hours thereafter. Then they start having difficulty in breathing.

What are the manifestations of this disease?

The baby's breathing becomes labored and grows progressively worse, until death from suffocation ensues in about one to three days.

What causes this condition?

The cause is unknown. Some believe it is due to inhalation of amniotic fluid (the fluid surrounding the baby in the womb) just before or at birth. Others believe it is due to a weak heart.

Does it invariably lead to death?

In almost every case.

What is the treatment for hyaline membrane disease?

Oxygen inhalations and increased moisture in the incubator.

Does the oxygen act in a harmful way in these cases, as in retrolental fibroplasia?

No, because the oxygen concentration is not high, and it is given only for a few days.

If an infant recovers from this condition, can it be normal?

Some babies have survived and are normal; others are permanently defective.

Is there any way to prevent this disease?

No.

EPIDEMIC DIARRHEA OF THE NEWBORN

What is epidemic diarrhea of the newborn?

It is a disease that occurs in hospital nurseries. Diarrhea is its most important feature, and, as its name implies, it occurs in epidemics. It is caused by a germ, the colon bacillus.

Is the bacillus coli germ normally present in the intestinal tract?

Yes. Some forms or strains are normally present, but certain other unusual strains produce this disease.

Can epidemic diarrhea of the newborn be caused by other germs?

Yes. Occasionally a virus or a staphylococcus can cause it.

Is this disease serious?

Yes.

Can it cause death?

Yes. Though now we have better ways of treating it than in former years.

Does this type of diarrhea occur in home deliveries?

No.

Is this condition different from other forms of diarrhea?

Yes, especially since it is limited to newborn babies.

Is this form of diarrhea contagious?

Yes.

What is the source of this germ in a nursery?

Usually an infant, or an adult carrier of this germ who works in or around the nursery.

Does epidemic diarrhea ever occur in older children?

Yes. It is sometimes found in children up to one year of age.

How is the disease diagnosed?

A culture is made from the stools.

What is the treatment for epidemic diarrhea of the newborn?

The antibiotics are effective in bringing this condition under control.

How long does it take to bring about a cure of this disease?

About one week.

Is it necessary to close a nursery when one case occurs?

Yes, and all the babies are treated prophylactically with antibiotics.

How can epidemic diarrhea be prevented?

By scrupulous cleanliness and avoidance of cross-infection.

Is there any vaccine to prevent this disease?

No.

After recovery, is any special care necessary for these infants?

Usually not.

DEHYDRATION FEVER

What is dehydration fever?

This condition occurs about the second or third day of the baby's life. His temperature rises to 101° or 103°, he is restless, irritable, cries a great deal, and loses weight.

What is the cause of dehydration fever?

The cause is not definitely known, but it is believed that dehydration fever is due to a temporary reduction in fluid intake.

How is this condition treated?

By giving fluids, either by mouth or under the skin. Within a day or two the temperature drops to normal and the baby recovers.

ATALECTASIS OF THE NEWBORN

What is atalectasis of the newborn?

This is a failure of expansion of some parts of the baby's lungs. These areas contain no air or oxygen and do not function properly.

What is the cause of atalectasis?

It may be due to obstruction by mucus or amniotic fluid in the respiratory passages, or it may be caused by an immaturity of the lung tissue with failure of this tissue to develop the ability to expand.

What are the manifestations of atalectasis?

The infant will have rapid, shallow breathing, may have a grunt while breathing, may become bluish because of lack of oxygen, and may display a pulling-in of the chest wall at its ribs and near the neck when attempting to breathe in.

Is there any way to make a definite diagnosis of this condition?

Examination of the chest will reveal that air is not entering certain parts of the lungs. In addition, an x-ray of the chest will show that air has not entered these areas.

What is the treatment for atalectasis of the newborn?

If there is any obstructive fluid in the respiratory passages, it must be sucked out. Sometimes, bronchoscopy is necessary in severe cases to remove any obstruction. In addition, the infant is kept in an incubator with high humidity and high oxygen content. It is important to stimulate the baby to breathe deeply by making it cry frequently, every few minutes, if necessary.

What is the outcome in these cases?

If the atalectasis is mild it will clear up in a few days with normal lung expansion. If it is extensive it may cause lack of oxygen to the brain and damage to the brain cells. In very severe cases, it may be fatal in one to two days.

HEMORRHAGIC DISEASE OF THE NEWBORN

What is hemorrhagic disease of the newborn?

This occurs about the second to fifth day of life, and is manifested by bleeding into the skin, the mucous membranes, the navel, and occasionally by bleeding from the rectum or vagina. There may be blood in the urine or in the vomitus.

What causes this type of hemorrhagic disease?

It is believed to be caused by a deficiency of one of the components in the blood-clotting mechanism, and by a deficiency of vitamin K.

What test is done to make a positive diagnosis?

The prothrombin clotting blood test is done. The clotting mechanism is found to be deficient in this condition.

What is the treatment for hemorrhagic disease of the newborn?

Vitamin K is given by injection into the vein or muscle. In severe cases, it is necessary to give a transfusion of fresh whole blood. This will promptly cure the condition.

Are there any permanent after-effects of this condition?

Usually not. Only in very rare, severe cases, where there may have been bleeding into the brain, will there be any serious after-effects.

How can this condition be prevented?

By giving a vitamin K injection to the newborn infant. This is done routinely for all premature babies and sometimes the mother is given vitamin K during her labor.

TETANY OF THE NEWBORN

What is tetany of the newborn?

It is a condition that occurs during the first week of life, associated with irritability, extreme restlessness, twitchings, and occasionally convulsions.

What causes tetany?

It is caused by a diminished amount of calcium in the blood. It may be brought on by impaired function of the parathyroid glands or the kidneys, or by feeding the child milk that has a higher proportion of phosphorus to calcium than is normal.

Does tetany occur in breast-fed infants?

It occurs less frequently in breast-fed than in bottle-fed infants because breast milk has the proper proportions of phosphorus and calcium.

What test can help to make a positive diagnosis?

A blood test for determination of the amount of calcium in the blood.

What is the treatment for tetany of the newborn?

Calcium solution is given intravenously, followed by the addition of a calcium-containing solution to the formula.

What can happen if the treatment is not given?

The infant will become more restless and will develop convulsions. These may be serious if calcium is not given quickly.

Can tetany be prevented?

Yes, by feeding breast milk, or by putting calcium into each bottle the infant takes.

SEPSIS OF THE NEWBORN

What is sepsis of the newborn?

It is a bloodstream infection or poisoning, occurring usually during the first week of life.

What is the cause of sepsis in newborns?

Bacteria entering the blood by way of the skin, mucous membranes, nose, mouth, or by way of the umbilicus.

Do these germs enter before birth or after birth?

The bacteria may enter the body at either time, and then gain access to the bloodstream.

What are the manifestations of this sepsis?

Failure to take feedings, vomiting, diarrhea, loss of weight, restlessness, high fever, and occasionally convulsions.

How can the diagnosis be established definitely?

Blood cultures are taken to determine whether bacteria are present in the bloodstream.

What is the treatment for sepsis of the newborn?

Prompt administration of the appropriate antibiotic in adequate doses.

Are there any complications of sepsis (blood poisoning)?

Yes. Pneumonia, meningitis, peritonitis, abscesses of various organs, or skin abscesses may appear.

What is the outlook in this condition?

With prompt and early recognition and treatment, the outlook is good. If not recognized early or if the infection is a severe, over-whelming one, it will lead to death of the infant within a short period of time.

Can sepsis be prevented?

If there is any evidence of infection in the mother before or during delivery, the baby should be given antibiotics prophylactically. If the baby shows any evidence of skin or navel infection, treatment with antibiotics should be instituted promptly.

THRUSH

What is thrush?

It is a disease of the tongue and mouth, usually occurring toward the end of the first week of life.

What is the cause of thrush?

It is caused by a fungus.

Where does this fungus come from?

Usually from the mother, who may have a mild fungus involvement of her vagina. During the birth passage the infant becomes infected with this same fungus. It takes about a week for the fungus to grow. It may also come from contamination by rubber nipples and other equipment that may have been in contact with another infant who has thrush.

What are the manifestations of thrush?

There is a heavy whitish coating on the tongue, which may spread to the gums, lips, and mucous membranes inside the mouth.

Is thrush serious?

No, and it is quite common.

What is the treatment for thrush?

Gentian violet is gently applied to the affected areas by rolling a cotton applicator over the tongue, gums, and mouth.

Does it take long to clear up thrush?

No. In about a week to ten days the condition will have cleared.

Can thrush be prevented?

If the mother is known to have a vaginal fungus infection with discharge, she should be treated for it during pregnancy.

In the nursery, should an infant with thrush be isolated?

Yes. In this way the spread from one infant to another can be prevented. The isolation should apply to all utensils used in the care of the infant.

OMPHALITIS

What is omphalitis?

It is an infection in the region of the navel (umbilicus) occurring during the first week of life.

Is omphalitis a serious infection?

Usually, it will clear promptly with adequate treatment. It may be serious if it spreads to a bloodstream infection.

What is the treatment for omphalitis?

a. Local applications to control the infection.
b. Antibiotics in adequate doses given internally.

CONGENITAL LARYNGEAL STRIDOR

What is congenital laryngeal stridor?

It is a noisy breathing, usually on inspiration, and especially pronounced with crying.

What is the cause of this condition?

It is usually caused by a flabbiness of the tissues around the larynx, particularly the epiglottis.

Are there ever any more serious causes for congenital laryngeal stridor?

Yes. In some cases there may be a malformation of the larynx or structures adjacent to it.

When is laryngeal stridor first noticed?

Usually at birth—and it may persist until the child is about twelve to eighteen months of age, when it gradually disappears.

Is any treatment necessary in the usual case of laryngeal stridor?

No. It is a self-limited condition. As the infant grows older the flabbiness of the laryngeal tissues disappears.

How are the more serious deformities in this region recognized?

By looking into the larynx with a laryngoscope. If the physician finds a cyst or web or other cause for obstruction, he will treat it at that time.

Is there need for special care in feeding infants with congenital laryngeal stridor?

Yes. These infants must be fed more slowly and carefully to prevent aspiration of the food into the windpipe. Sometimes, these babies may find difficulty in sucking from a nipple and may need spoon-feeding.

Is the usual case of laryngeal stridor serious?

No. It may sound very annoying to the parents, but it is usually not serious. It is important that the parents be reassured that the condition will eventually clear up spontaneously.

30 *Infant Feeding and Bowel Function*

BREAST FEEDING

Is breast feeding preferable to bottle feeding?

Yes.

Why is breast milk best for the newborn child?

It has all the proper elements for the baby's best growth and development; it is clean and sterile; it is of the proper temperature. Also, immune substances are contained in mother's milk which help protect the newborn child against disease.

Are there psychological advantages to nursing?

Yes, for both the mother and the child. The closeness, the cuddling, etc., are important for both the baby and the mother.

Does a nursing mother require any special diet?

She may eat a full diet, being sure to include approximately a quart of milk a day. She should take plenty of fluids and she should be sure to include eggs, meat, fruits, vegetables, and cereal.

Should the nursing mother avoid certain foods?

Yes. She should avoid gassy foods such as cabbage and rhubarb, and also excessive amounts of chocolate.

Should a nursing mother supplement her diet with vitamins?

Only if she has a vitamin deficiency or fails to eat a full well-balanced diet.

Do drugs or medications that the mother takes affect her milk?

Consult your physician on this matter. Most medicines do not show up in the mother's milk, but some may affect the baby.

What general precautions should the nursing mother take?

She should:

a. Get plenty of rest.

b. Get plenty of relaxation.

c. Avoid tensions and anxieties.

d. Avoid excessive smoking.

e. Avoid excessive drinking of alcoholic beverages.

Will nursing adversely affect the mother's teeth?

No. However, she should take an adequate supply of calcium in her diet every day. This will be accomplished by drinking sufficient milk.

Is nursing ever harmful to the mother?

Yes, if she is emotionally disturbed by the act. Those women who become tense or who find nursing exceedingly disagreeable should not be forced to nurse.

If the mother is ill or has a chronic debilitating disease, should she nurse?

No.

When is it wisest not to breast feed a child?

When the child is very small or weak, or is premature, or has a cleft palate or harelip.

How soon after birth can nursing be started?

The very first day.

Is there any milk in the mother's breast during the first few days after delivery?

No, but the nursing child does obtain a substance known as colostrum.

What is colostrum, and what is its value?

Colostrum is a substance which is secreted by the breasts before the milk fully comes in. It contains many immune substances which may help to protect the baby during its first few days of life.

Does the nursing child obtain sufficient nourishment the first two or three days of life, before breast milk begins to flow?

Yes. The breast feeding is often supplemented by bottle feeding.

When does real milk start to flow?

About the third or fourth day after birth.

What starts the flow of milk into the mother's breast?

Certain hormones in the mother's body. Also, the baby's sucking will accelerate the flow of milk.

At what intervals should the baby breast feed?

Normal healthy babies may nurse every three to four hours.

If the baby seems to need it, is it permissible to nurse more often?

Yes, but not more often than every two hours.

Should the baby nurse on one or both breasts?

In general, it is best to nurse at both breasts. Later on, it may be wiser to alternate breasts at different feedings.

How long should each nursing last?

About twenty minutes. Sometimes, it is better to allow the child ten to fifteen minutes at each breast.

What should be done if the baby falls asleep during nursing?

Gentle stimulation may help to wake him. He should be permitted a rest of five minutes during nursing but not longer. Following such a rest, he may resume sucking at a normal rate.

In what position should the mother nurse the baby?

During the first few days, while in the hospital, she may nurse while lying on her side, in bed. Later, it is better to nurse while sitting in a comfortable chair.

Should water be given to the baby between nursings?

This is not necessary in most instances, but if the baby seems to be thirsty and cries, he may be given a few ounces of boiled water.

Is it permissible to skip nursings if the child has not awakened?

Within the first few days, it is best not to skip nursings. Later on, the baby may be permitted a longer sleep and have a bottle to substitute for a nursing during the middle of the night.

What is the treatment for "cracked" nipples?

A mother with cracked nipples should skip a few nursings, or alternate the breasts. The use of a nipple shield helps to protect the breast and helps it to heal more quickly. A soothing ointment may be applied after each nursing, but it must be washed off before the baby is again put to the breast.

What special care should be given the nipples?

Cleanliness is the most important objective. The nipples should be washed before and after each nursing. A comfortable, well-fitting uplift brassière should be worn.

What is the treatment for "caked" breasts?

The nursings should be stopped until the condition has healed.

Should nursing be stopped if an infection of the breast occurs?

Yes.

If it is necessary to stop nursing because of a breast condition, can nursing be resumed at a later date?

Yes, in most instances. However, in certain cases it is wiser to stop nursing permanently and switch to bottle feeding.

How long should breast nursing be continued?

Approximately four to seven months.

Can a woman stop breast feeding after three to four months?

Yes.

Is weaning a difficult process?

No. Most babies are given a supplementary bottle during the early months of life and therefore will not resist the change to bottle feeding later on.

How soon can a supplementary bottle be started?

When the child is two to three weeks old. When the child is two months old it is often wise to skip two nursings a day and replace them with bottles.

What can be done if the mother must be away from the child for two or three days?

The breasts can be pumped so that the milk supply will not diminish. This will enable the mother to resume nursing when she returns.

If the mother and child are to be separated for more than a few days, is it wiser to discontinue nursing completely and to start bottle feeding?

Yes.

Is sudden, abrupt weaning harmful?

No. Most children take the change from breast feeding to bottle feeding without difficulty.

Are vitamins and solid foods given to children who are breast-fed, just as they are given to bottle-fed children?

Yes. There is no variation in these supplementary substances.

What does the mother do when she stops nursing?

She usually wears a tight breast binder or brassière. It is also advisable to limit her intake of fluids for several days. If breasts are not emptied periodically they will not refill. The baby's sucking and breast emptying are the greatest impetus to milk formation.

Is it permissible for the mother to take pain-relieving medications when she stops nursing?

Yes.

BOTTLE FEEDING

If the mother cannot nurse, is bottle feeding almost as satisfactory?

Yes. There are many excellent preparations of formulas which give the newborn child all that he needs in the way of nourishment.

How soon after birth can a child start getting his formula?

Within eight to twelve hours.

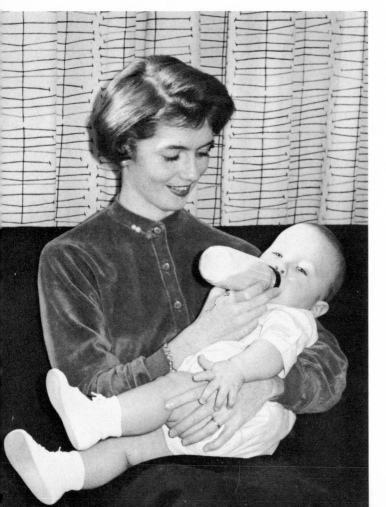

Bottle Feeding. This photograph shows one of the approved positions for holding a child while being bottle fed. However, there are many other approved positions, including allowing the child to lie flat on his back or side. Many pediatricians feel that the child derives great comfort by being held in his parent's arms while being fed.

How much formula is given at first?

About a half-ounce during the first day, increased to an ounce at each feeding the second day, one and a half to two ounces on the third day, and increased gradually as the baby needs it thereafter.

How can a mother know what equipment is needed to prepare a formula?

Your child specialist (pediatrician) will supply you with this information. Also, many hospitals give lectures to mothers about formula preparation before they leave the hospital.

From whom will a mother receive instructions about methods of sterilization?

a. From your pediatrician or physician.
b. From your hospital.
c. From the baby's nurse or from a nursing agency.

What types of bottles and nipples should be used?

There are many excellent ones on the market. It makes very little difference what you use, as long as it functions well. The small or large nipples are equally effective.

Is it safe to use plastic bottles?

Yes, if they can be sterilized adequately.

How can a mother tell if the nipple is good?

Turn the bottle upside down; the milk should come through the nipple openings freely, a drop at a time.

Is it permissible to enlarge nipple openings?

Yes, with a sterile needle.

What should be done if too much milk flows through the nipple?

Discard that nipple and use another one.

What are the basic ingredients of most baby formulas?

Most formulas are prepared with evaporated milk, water, and some

663

form of additional carbohydrate, usually dextrimaltose. Some physicians prefer that a mixture of homogenized milk be used instead of evaporated milk. There are also many preparations on the market, in either liquid or powder form, which require merely the addition of water. All of these various preparations can be used effectively and safely in infant feeding.

What proportions of the various ingredients are used in the formulas?

In the evaporated milk formulas, there are usually eight ounces of evaporated milk, sixteen ounces of boiled water, and three tablespoons of dextrimaltose or two tablespoons of Karo syrup or granulated sugar. This is divided into six or seven bottles of three and a half to four ounces each. This is the formula most widely used when the baby first leaves the hospital.

Does the formula vary as the child grows older?

Yes. The proportion of evaporated milk is gradually increased, until finally the child is receiving thirteen ounces of evaporated milk, nineteen ounces of boiled water, and four tablespoons of dextrimaltose.

Does this last formula need to be changed often?

No. These proportions can usually remain fixed until the child is ready for whole milk.

When can the formula be changed to whole milk?

When the child is about five to seven months of age.

Is it necessary to add any other substances to the prepared formulas?

No. They are usually made with adequate amounts of all necessary ingredients. Also, these preparations come with complete and simple instructions.

Can it harm the baby if the proportions of the various ingredients are varied slightly?

No.

Is it safe to use homogenized milk or approved milk in making a formula?

Yes.

What is the best method of changing from one formula to another?

This should be done gradually, unless the first formula definitely does not agree with the baby.

In changing from an evaporated milk formula to whole milk, it is advisable to reduce all the components in the formula while replacing them with whole milk, as follows:

Formula	1st Week	2nd Week	3rd Week	4th Week
Evaporated milk	10 oz.	7 oz.	4 oz.	0
Boiled water	14 oz.	9 oz.	4 oz.	0
Dextrimaltose No. 1	3 tbls.	2 tbls.	1 tbls.	0
Homogenized milk	8 oz.	16 oz.	24 oz.	32 oz.

How many bottles are made in the formula?

In the beginning, divide the formula into six or seven bottles of three and a half to four ounces each. Later, four to six ounces are put into each bottle. As the baby grows older and takes fewer feedings, the thirty-two-ounce formula may be divided into five bottles.

How often should a baby be given his bottle?

Some babies can go on a four-hour schedule from birth. Smaller babies may require a three-hour schedule during the daytime and a four-hour schedule at night, making seven feedings in a twenty-four-hour period.

Should the baby be made to adhere to a rigid feeding schedule?

No, especially in the beginning. It is best to feed the baby as often as he needs it. This is called the "self-demand schedule." As he grows older, he will adopt a more definite pattern, usually of four-hour intervals.

What should be done if the baby wants to be fed every two hours?

Let the baby have his formula every two hours.

How soon after birth do children start regulating their own schedule?

Most babies will develop a fairly regular four-hour schedule at about four to six weeks of age, some a little earlier, some a little later.

Should a baby be forced into a rigid schedule?

No. Let the baby, within reason, decide his own schedule. Gentle persuasion into a regular schedule can be carried out, however. Much will depend on the mother's time schedule as well as on the baby's requirement.

Should the baby be awakened for a night feeding?

In general, no. Sometimes, it may be wise to wake him in order to help him into a more regular schedule.

Is there any harm in letting the baby's feedings go beyond the four-hour interval?

No.

Should the baby be awakened for a night feeding?

No. It is preferable to wait until he awakens. However, if the baby tends to awaken at an inopportune hour, such as 4 or 5 A.M., it may be wiser to awaken him earlier. Some mothers find it best to wake the baby at 11 to 12 P.M. while they are still awake, so that the baby will sleep through until 6 or 7 A.M.

How soon do most babies skip their night feedings?

Many babies skip the 2 A.M. feeding when they reach two to three months of age. There are great variations, all of which fall into the category of normal.

What are the best hours for feeding the baby?

This depends on the family pattern of living. Some babies will thrive on a 6 A.M., 10 A.M., 2 P.M., 6 P.M., 10 P.M., 2 A.M. schedule. In other families the hours can be varied to 7 A.M., 11 A.M., 3 P.M., etc.

How much of the formula should the baby take?

This will vary according to each baby's needs. In the early months, he will take two to four ounces, later on four to six ounces, and still later six to eight ounces at each feeding. The average total daily intake during the first month of life will be twenty to twenty-five ounces; later, it increases to twenty-five to thirty-two ounces, and in some instances the baby may require as much as forty ounces of formula. As solid foods are added, most babies will take less formula.

Do most babies take the same amount at each feeding?

No. There may be great variations from feeding to feeding.

Should each bottle contain the same amount of formula?

Yes. However, it is usually best to let the baby set his own pattern, as he may develop the habit of taking more at one feeding than at another.

Should the baby be expected to drain each bottle?

No.

Can the amounts in the bottles be varied?

Yes, if the mother gets to know how much the baby takes at certain feedings.

What should be done with milk that the baby does not take?

Discard it.

What should be done when the baby takes only an ounce of milk at one feeding and wants more an hour later?

For a time, it is permissible to allow this habit to develop. In such instances, the formula should be put into the refrigerator and re-warmed for the remainder of the feedings.

How long should it take for a baby to drain his bottle?

Most babies will fulfill their requirements within ten to fifteen minutes. If the baby dawdles, discard the remainder of the bottle, for he has probably finished feeding.

667

Should a baby be permitted to spend an hour at his feeding?

No. Some babies develop the dawdling habit; this should be discouraged.

Should the baby be permitted to cry for his feeding if he awakens too early?

On the self-demand schedule the baby is usually permitted to eat whenever he wishes. However, sometimes it is necessary to vary that procedure, and it does no harm to permit a baby to cry for a little while before he gets his feeding. It is never necessary to rush to feed the baby when he cries. It should also be remembered that sometimes he may only want water.

Should babies be given water between feedings?

Yes. One to three ounces of boiled water may be given once or twice a day between feedings. It should not be forced upon those children who reject it.

Do babies often take too much of their formula?

In general, babies stop when they are satisfied. Occasionally, a baby will take too much and will usually vomit the excess. There is no harm in this.

When are vitamins added to the diet?

At about four to six weeks of age.

What vitamin preparations are usually used?

A multivitamin drop, usually one that contains vitamins A, B_1, B_2, B_6, B_{12}, C, D, and E. Most vitamin preparations on the market contain all of these vitamins.

How are these vitamins given?

Practically all of these preparations are soluble in water, milk, or fruit juices. They can either be dissolved in these liquids or they may be dropped directly on the infant's tongue.

How much of the vitamins is given?

Start with one to three drops for the first few days and then increase gradually up to fifteen drops a day. Most vitamins come with medicine droppers which are marked with accurate instructions on how much to give.

Can the droppers hurt the baby's tongue?

No. Today most droppers are made of plastic material.

What is the maximum amount of vitamins to be given each day?

Fifteen drops or 0.6 cc. This amount should be given every day.

Should vitamins be given in the summertime?

Yes, in the same amounts as during other months.

Is there any great harm if the child doesn't finish the bottle into which the vitamins have been dissolved?

It is not harmful if the child skips an occasional feeding in which the vitamins are given.

Do vitamins exist naturally in milk?

Yes. All evaporated milk contains an adequate supply of vitamin D to prevent rickets. Some of the prepared formulas also have vitamins C and D added.

Is it possible to give too much of a particular vitamin?

Not ordinarily. There is a great deal of leeway in the amount the body can tolerate. However, on occasion an excess has been given with harmful results. This is a rare occurrence.

Can the vitamins occasionally cause a rash?

Yes.

What is done for rashes caused by vitamins?

It may be necesary to stop giving the vitamins entirely for a while or to substitute a preparation containing only vitamins A, C, and D. Some physicians prefer to start with an A, C, D preparation.

At what age is orange juice started?

Usually at about two months of age.

How is orange juice given?

Start with one teaspoonful, dilute it with an equal quantity of boiled water. Increase gradually up to one ounce each of juice and water.

Is it necessary to use fresh orange juice?

No. The frozen or canned orange juice is adequate.

Do all babies tolerate orange juice?

No. Some babies will vomit or develop a rash from orange juice. In that event, do not give it.

Is there any harm if the baby does not tolerate orange juice?

Not if the baby is getting a multivitamin preparation containing vitamin C.

Can juices other than orange juice be added?

Yes, but be sure they have an adequate supply of vitamin C.

Can cod liver oil be given instead of vitamin drops?

Yes, but only to supply vitamins A and D. In that case, it is essential to add vitamin C in the form of orange juice or special vitamin C drops.

Can various fish liver oil preparations be used?

Yes, but again it is necessary to add vitamin C.

Is it necessary to add vitamin B when giving drops other than the multivitamin preparations?

Yes. It is advisable to add a vitamin B preparation when using cod liver oil or fish liver oil only.

When may the baby be given solid foods?

When he is about two months of age. Some physicians start the baby on solid foods a little earlier, some a little later.

Which solids are given first?

Either cereal or fruit. Rice or barley cereals are excellent too. Applesauce and mashed ripe banana are also frequently given as first foods.

How much of these foods is given?

Always start with one teaspoonful of a new food and increase the amount gradually, depending on how well the baby takes to it, until about half a jar or several tablespoons of each food can be given.

Should solid foods be given before or after the formula?

In the beginning, it may be necessary to give a few ounces of the formula first and then introduce the solid food. Later on, it is better to give the solid food first and allow the baby to take the milk later.

At what feeding should the solids be given?

This does not matter. In general, cereal may be given at the 10 A.M. and 6 P.M. feedings; fruit at the 2 P.M. feeding. This can be varied at will.

Do all babies readily take solid food?

No. If the baby spits out the solid food, try it again and again, until he gets used to it. If the baby definitely cannot manage solid foods, stop the attempts at giving them for a week or two, and then start over.

How should solids be fed?

With a small spoon.

Can solids ever be given through a bottle?

If necessary, by cutting off the tip of the nipple.

What cooked cereals can be used?

Farina, Cream of Wheat, or oatmeal may be used well cooked. This usually means cooking for twenty to thirty minutes. Precooked cereals now on the market are much easier for the mother to prepare.

When can any cereal be given?

At two to four months of age.

Can prepared fruits out of cans be given?

Yes. These preparations are all adequate.

How are solids usually added to diets?

This varies widely according to each physician's custom and also according to the child's individual taste. The following schedule is often utilized:

Age	Add
2 mos.	Cereals (barley and rice). Fruits (applesauce and mashed banana).
3 mos.	Other cereals and fruits.
4 mos.	Vegetables (carrots, peas, green beans, squash). Baby soups (chicken, vegetable, tomato). Fruit combinations.
5 mos.	All vegetables, including baked potato. All baby soups and vegetable combinations. Egg yolk (coddled, hard-boiled, or in baby cans).
6 mos.	Strained baby meats (beef, beef liver, beef heart mashed, broiled chicken liver). Jello, junket.
7 mos.	All strained baby meats, custard, chocolate pudding, whole egg (yolk and white).

What are good diets for children of 8, 10, 12, and 24 months of age?

DIET SCHEDULE FOR BABY:
8 MONTHS OLD

ON ARISING:

Vitamin drops and orange juice.

BREAKFAST:

   Cereal—any cooked or precooked cereal with milk.

   Egg—coddled, soft-boiled, or hard-boiled.

   Bottle.

NOON MEAL:

   Vegetables—all prepared, strained vegetables or combinations.
      Fresh vegetables, cooked and strained.
      Potato, baked or boiled with butter added.

   Meats—chicken liver, broiled and mashed or strained.
      Chicken, minced or shredded.
      Beefsteak patty, finely ground and broiled.
      All strained meats.

   Desserts—any prepared fruits or fruit combinations.

   Bottle—if baby wants it.

3:30 P.M.

   Bottle, with arrowroot cracker or cookie. (Some babies prefer a
   morning bottle on arising. In that case give vitamin drops and
   orange juice at this time.)

EVENING MEAL:

   Cereal—as at morning meal—or
      Baby soup—any of the prepared baby soups, mixed with a little
      milk.

   Egg—if not given in the morning.

   Dessert—banana or any of the baby fruit combinations, with a
      little milk or cream. Jello, junket, custard, chocolate or tapioca
      pudding.

   Bottle.

NOTE: The baby may not take all these foods. This is a menu from
   which to select the foods. Do not insist upon giving the baby any
   food not desired.

NEW FOODS THAT MAY BE ADDED TO DIET LIST: AT 10 MONTHS

STARCHY FOODS:

Spaghetti, noodles, pastina
(these may be well cooked and strained).

Rice, sweet potato.

CREAM:

Sweet or sour cream.

CHEESE:

Cream cheese, cottage or pot cheese
(may be mixed with a little cream or milk).

BACON:

Crisp.

JUICES:

Other fruit juices, in addition to orange juice.

NOTE: At this age, the baby may refuse certain foods, or may refuse milk. This is not unusual. He may even go on jags—all milk, no solids, or the reverse, for periods. Do not be disturbed by this.

DIET LIST: ONE YEAR OLD

BREAKFAST:

Any cooked or precooked cereal with milk.

Egg—coddled, poached, soft-boiled, or hard-boiled.

Strip of bacon may be added.

Bread or toast. Milk.

Vitamin drops and orange juice may be given during the morning or at mealtime.

NOON MEAL:

Meats—chicken, chicken liver, calf's liver, lamb chop, lamb stew, beefsteak patty, chopped meats.

Fish—broiled or boiled. No mackerel, salmon, or salty fish.

Vegetables—all the prepared, strained vegetables or combinations of them. Strained, cooked fresh vegetables. When the baby is ready for chopped foods, these may be used.

Dessert—all prepared baby fruit desserts.

MIDAFTERNOON:

Milk with crackers, cookies, or toast and butter.

EVENING MEAL:

Any one of the baby soups, plain or creamed.

Spaghetti, noodles, or pastina.

Cheese—cream, cottage, or pot cheese. Sweet or sour cream.

Raw vegetables—chopped carrot or tomato.

Dessert—banana and sweet cream, junket, Jello, custard, chocolate or tapioca pudding; or fruit desserts.

Milk.

Occasionally egg or cereal may be omitted from the morning meal and given in the evening. Other fruit juices may be substituted for orange juice.

DO NOT FORCE THE BABY TO TAKE ANY FOOD OR MILK NOT DESIRED.

DIET LIST: TWO YEARS OLD

BREAKFAST:

Fruit—orange, grapefruit, apple, prunes, cooked pears, peaches, or apricots; or any fruit juice.

Cereal—any cooked or dry cereal, with milk or cream.

Eggs—may be given in any form. Bacon may be added.

Bread or toast and butter.

DIET LIST: TWO YEARS OLD

NOON MEAL:

Soup—any clear broth or creamed vegetable soup.

Meat—chicken or chicken liver; beef or calf's liver; lamb chop or lamb stew; ground beefsteak patty or roast beef; diced meats.

Fish—any fresh fish, broiled, baked, or boiled.

Vegetables—all cooked vegetables—preferably fresh or frozen. Prepared, chopped vegetables may be used. Raw vegetables occasionally.

Potato, rice, spaghetti, macaroni, or pastina.

Dessert—any raw or cooked fruit, custard, junket, Jello, puddings, ice cream.

MIDAFTERNOON:

Milk with crackers, cookies, or toast and jam.

EVENING MEAL:

Any fruit or vegetable juice, or soup if not given at noon.

Salad of cooked or raw vegetables.

Cheese—cream, cottage, pot, Swiss, or American.

Sour cream.

Spaghetti or noodles.

Eggs—if not given at breakfast.

Dessert—banana or berries and cream, or other desserts as listed above.

Bread and butter. Milk.

NOTE: The vitamin drops may be given at any mealtime.

Do not give any fried or canned fish; no salted, pickled, or smoked foods; no highly seasoned sauces or gravies; no pastries or rich cakes.

The above list does not represent all the foods that must be given.

It is only a suggested list from which to start the menu for the day.

NEVER FORCE THE CHILD TO EAT ANY FOOD OR TO DRINK MILK.

Is it harmful if the baby tends to take too much solid food and cuts down on his liquids?

No. It is common for the child to drink less formula or milk as he takes more solids. This will vary from child to child.

Does the amount of solids in the formula the child takes vary from day to day?

Yes.

How should new foods be introduced into the diet?

Always try to introduce one new food at a time. Always start new foods with a very small amount and increase gradually on successive days.

Can babies eat the foods safely from a jar or can?

Yes. Foods as they are processed today do not spoil as long as the container is unopened.

How long can leftover foods in a jar or can be used?

After opening, they can be kept in a refrigerator for about a day or two without spoiling.

Is it necessary to use canned foods?

No. Many mothers prefer to prepare their own fruits, vegetables, soups, or meats. They should be well cooked, and well puréed, and put through a strainer so that they may be digested easily.

Can small amounts of salt or sugar be added to the foods for seasoning purposes?

Yes.

Which should be the heaviest meal of the day?

Preferably, the noon meal.

When can the child be permitted to feed himself?

Some babies will start finger-feeding at nine to eleven months of age. This may be quite messy but the child should be allowed to do it. It represents a step toward self-sufficiency.

When are chopped or junior foods introduced into the diet?

When the baby is about ten to twelve months of age.

When should cup training be started?

When the baby is about ten to twelve months of age.

When can the bottle be eliminated?

Babies vary a great deal in this matter, as they do in all feeding matters. Some will allow themselves to be fed from a cup at twelve to fifteen months of age. Others will take juice from a cup but insist upon milk from a bottle until eighteen months of age. Do not be insistent in eliminating the bottle. Some children may require a bottle until two years of age. This will do no harm.

When can sterilization of bottles and nipples be stopped?

It is best to continue sterilization until the baby is nine months of age. Thereafter, the bottles may be washed thoroughly with soap and hot water, but the nipples should be sterilized for a longer period.

How should the baby be held during feeding?

It is best to hold him in a semi-erect position in the curve of your arm. In this way, the air bubble he swallows during feeding will rise to the top of his stomach and will come up as a "burp" more easily. In addition, the baby will not bring up any of the milk with the burp.

Is it permissible to feed the baby in a semi-erect position on a small pillow?

Yes.

Is it permissible to feed the baby lying down?

Yes, but he should be picked up once or twice during the feeding to bring up the air bubble.

What can be done to help the baby bring up the air bubble?

The mother puts him over her shoulder and holds him there for several minutes. Sometimes, stroking his back or gently patting him will help.

How soon after feeding can the baby be put down in a lying position?

It is best to keep him upright for ten to fifteen minutes after a feeding.

At what age can the child be fed in a highchair?

When he is able to sit up comfortably for about ten to fifteen minutes. This will be somewhere between four and six months of age.

What is the significance of hiccups?

They are spasms of the diaphragm and have no special significance. They occur normally.

What should be done for hiccups?

In most cases, nothing should be done. A small drink of water may help to end them more quickly.

Is it normal for infants to spit up or regurgitate some of their feedings?

Yes. "Burping" often brings up a little of the formula. It may occur from changing the child's position or when he is taking a little too much food.

Is vomiting serious?

Occasional vomiting is not serious. It may be caused by the same factors that cause slight regurgitation. Repeated or persistent vomiting should lead you to consult your physician.

COLIC

What is colic?

It is a pain in the baby's abdomen due to spasm of the intestines.

What are the symptoms of colic?

Excessive crying, especially in the evening hours, and drawing up of the child's legs, as if he is in pain; sometimes these symptoms are accompanied by extreme irritability.

What causes colic?

There are many conditions that lead to it. Among them are:

a. Underfeeding and hunger.
b. Excessive carbohydrate in the formula.
c. Too much butterfat in the formula.
d. Swallowing air and failure to burp.
e. Allergy to cow's milk.
f. Immaturity of the baby's nervous system.
g. Tenseness and anxiety in the home.
h. The mother's insecurity and fear of handling the baby.
i. Improper feeding technique.
j. Fatigue.

How is colic prevented?

By finding out which of the above factors is the cause and by correcting it. It is often necessary to obtain the doctor's help in this matter.

What is the first-aid treatment when the child is crying with severe colicky pain?

Be calm. Hold the baby erect, close to your body, and keep something warm near his abdomen. (Do not burn him with a hot-water bottle.) If advised by your doctor, a small enema may help him to expel gas and thus relieve the colic. Placing the child on his abdomen on a warm pad may also help to relieve the colic.

Should medicines for colic be given without a doctor's advice?

Never.

How long does colic last?

Some babies have colic for two to three months, and then it disappears spontaneously.

Are second and third children in the family less colicky?

Yes, because of the greater experience of the mother in handling them.

Is colic dangerous?

No.

BOWEL MOVEMENTS

How many bowel movements a day are normal for a newborn child?

Anywhere from one to five movements a day. Breast-fed babies may have more bowel movements than bottle-fed infants. Occasionally, the baby will have a movement with each feeding. As long as the consistency of the stool is good, the number of stools per day does not matter too much.

What is the normal consistency of stools?

They should be mushy or pasty, or even somewhat firmer. They should have a fairly sweetish odor.

What is the normal color of an infant's stool?

Golden yellow. It may also be greenish or turn greenish-brown after standing for some time. This is normal.

Is constipation serious?

Ordinarily not. If the baby has one firm stool per day, nothing need be done about it as long as the infant is not uncomfortable.

Is it normal for some infants to strain at stool?

Yes. This will disappear as the child grows older, unless he is unusually constipated.

Can the mother help the child when he is straining at stool?

Yes. Flexing the legs on the abdomen frequently helps.

Should suppositories be given if the baby is constipated?

Only on the doctor's advice.

Is it ever necessary to stretch the anus when children are constipated?

Occasionally, yes. However, in most cases the bowel movement itself acts to stretch the anal opening.

Are there ever a few streaks of blood in a constipated stool?

Yes. The hard stool stretches the anal opening and may cause a small scratch on the surface. This in itself is not serious. This can often be helped by a suppository or by making the stool softer.

How can the stools be made softer?

a. Increase the baby's water intake.
b. Increase the carbohydrates added to the formula.
c. If boiled milk is being used, reduce or eliminate the boiling.
d. Reduce constipating foods, such as banana, Jello, junket, chocolate, cheese.
e. Increase laxative foods, such as cooked fruits, cooked vegetables.
f. Give prune juice or cooked prunes.

Can mineral oil ever be given to soften the stools?

Yes, but only on a doctor's prescription.

Are there any other medications which can soften the child's stool?

There are many medicines on the market which will perform this function, but they must be given only on a doctor's prescription.

Is it permissible to use laxatives to soften the stool?

Usually not. The eagerness to remedy constipation may produce a diarrhea in a baby. This is a much more serious condition and a much more difficult one to control.

DIARRHEA

What is diarrhea?

Too frequent stools. In an infant this may mean ten to twelve or fifteen per day.

Is the character and color of the stools usually changed in infant diarrhea?

Yes. The stools may show undigested material and may be greenish or greenish-brown in color and may have a foul odor.

Are diarrheal stools irritating to the child?

Yes. They may cause a rash on the buttocks.

What is the significance of blood or mucus in the stools?

The appearance of blood or mucus is due to prolonged irritation of the mucous membrane lining of the intestinal tract and is an indication that the child needs medical treatment.

What are the causes of infant diarrhea?

a. Faulty technique in preparation of the formula.
b. Excessive carbohydrates in the formula.
c. Allergy to cow's milk.
d. Introduction of a new food which is irritating.
e. Excessive amounts of laxative foods.
f. Infection within the intestinal tract.
g. Infection elsewhere within the body.

How long does diarrhea last?

It may be a very short-lived temporary digestive upset or it may persist for some time and be a symptom of a more serious general condition.

What is the treatment for infant diarrhea?

a. Skip one or two feedings to give the intestinal tract a rest.
b. Give only boiled water or weak tea in small amounts until feedings are resumed.
c. Start feedings with more dilute formulas, preferably with less carbohydrate and fat.
d. Give smaller amounts during the first few feedings, perhaps only one to two ounces per feeding for a day or two. Supplement the lack of formula with boiled water.

e. Add a bland constipating food such as mashed ripe banana, raw scraped apple, and a little pot cheese which has been thinned with boiled water.

Can paregoric or other medicines be used to stop diarrhea?

These medications should be given only under a doctor's direction.

Should a laxative be given to stop diarrhea?

No. This is incorrect treatment.

When can a normal diet be resumed after an attack of diarrhea?

When the child has had several hard, firm movements for a period of two to three days. At first, small amounts of the baby's normal diet should be given, and then the amounts should be increased gradually.

Can milk be resumed after a diarrhea?

If the baby has been on a formula, the formula should be resumed gradually. If he has been on whole milk, use diluted boiled milk until his stools have returned to normal. Slowly return to full-strength unboiled milk, if that is what the baby was taking prior to the diarrhea.

What should be done if the diarrhea is persistent and severe?

Contact your physician and get instructions from him. Stop all feedings until he arrives.

Is vomiting serious when associated with diarrhea?

Yes. The baby will then lose fluids and minerals from his body tissues which must be replaced quickly.

Do cases of diarrhea have to be treated in the hospital?

Serious cases should be; mild cases may be treated at home.

What treatment is carried out in the hospital for severe cases of diarrhea?

Oral feedings are discontinued and the baby is given the proper amounts of nourishment and fluids through the veins.

What is the outlook for severe cases of infant diarrhea?

If treated early in their course, practically all cases recover. The serious cases and deaths from infant diarrhea that used to occur many years ago are now a thing of the past, owing to improved methods of treatment.

Were these cases of diarrhea once called "summer complaint" or "summer diarrhea"?

Yes.

For how long a period is hospitalization necessary in a case of severe infant diarrhea?

Approximately seven to ten days. The child must be hospitalized until the diarrhea and vomiting have stopped, the infection has cleared up, and the infant has returned to his normal diet schedule.

Are special formulas used for diarrheas?

Yes. In some cases, the infant is not put back on his original formula but is given a new formula containing skimmed milk or a fat-free mixture. Some physicians may prescribe a lactic acid mixture in the formula, or a high-protein formula.

How long are these special formulas continued after an attack of diarrhea?

For several weeks.

Are episodes of diarrhea ever recurrent?

Occasionally. In these instances, it is necessary to find the underlying cause and treat it strenuously.

What are the common causes for recurrent diarrhea?

a. An allergy.

b. An infection in the intestinal tract.

c. A form of celiac disease. (See Chapter 29, on Infant and Childhood Diseases.)

d. An abnormality within the intestinal tract.

Is allergy to cow's milk a common condition among children?

A very small percentage of children cannot take cow's milk because they are allergic to it.

How can one tell if an infant is allergic to cow's milk?

Usually there will be vomiting, colicky pains, loose stools, or mucus in the stools. Occasionally, there will be a rash, particularly on the face. There may also be failure to gain weight, or actual weight loss.

Is there often a history of allergy in the family of a child who is allergic to cow's milk?

Yes. A careful history will often reveal another member of the family with a food allergy.

What is the treatment for an allergy to cow's milk?

Do not give the child cow's milk.

What substitutes may be used for cow's milk?

Goat's milk, or a prepared synthetic milk produced from soybean.

Are these substitutes for milk satisfactory?

Yes. They contain all the elements necessary for the infant's growth and development.

Should other milk products be excluded from the diet of an allergic baby?

Yes. Cheeses, butter, etc., should not be given.

Can a child allergic to cow's milk ever take milk?

Yes. Usually, after the child is a year or eighteen months of age, he will lose this allergy and can then be put back on regular milk. This must be done slowly after testing the child with small amounts.

When the child is allergic to cow's milk, should vitamins and juices be given?

Yes. These are added in the usual way.

If a child is allergic to cow's milk, is it possible that he will demonstrate other allergies?

Yes. For this reason, it is important to be cautious in adding any new food to the diet of such an infant.

Can allergy to milk be a serious condition in children?

There are occasional children who may go into collapse when given cow's milk. In such a case, make sure to avoid giving cow's milk again.

31

Infectious and Virus Diseases

What are the causes of infectious diseases, and what are examples of each?

   a. Bacteria (typhoid fever, pneumonia, etc.).

   b. Protozoa (amebic dysentery, malaria).

   c. Rickettsia (typhus fever, rocky mountain spotted fever).

   d. Virus (influenza, smallpox, measles).

   e. Fungus (athlete's foot, blastomycosis).

What is the difference between bacteria and viruses?

Bacteria may be seen under the ordinary microscope; viruses are too small to be seen except under a very high-powered electron microscope. Bacteria are too large to pass through certain earthenware filters, whereas viruses are small enough to pass through these filters.

Do bacteria and viruses require living cells for their growth and multiplication?

Bacteria do not. They can be grown, and they multiply, on nonliving substances; viruses, however, cannot grow or multiply except in the presence of living tissue cells, either animal or human.

How are viral diseases spread?

By contact, by droplet infection in the air, and by intermediates (vectors) such as mosquitoes, lice, ticks, etc.

Do bacteria and viruses respond to antibiotic and chemical agents in the same manner?

No. Many bacteria are killed or inactivated by the antibiotic and chemotherapeutic drugs (penicillin, the mycin group, the sulfa group, etc.), but viruses are not so affected.

Does one attack of a virus disease protect the individual against further attack?

Not always. In many instances, as in smallpox, measles, polio, etc., this does hold true. But there are other diseases, such as the common cold, influenza, etc., which can occur many times in the same person.

How can immunity against virus diseases be obtained?

By the development and use of vaccines made from dead or weakened viruses. Poliomyelitis and influenza vaccines are examples. Other viral vaccines are being developed as greater success in growing the pure viruses is achieved.

Is there an effective vaccine for the common cold?

Not as yet. Recent work, however, seems to hold hope for the future development of such a vaccine.

TYPHOID FEVER

What is typhoid fever, and how is it transmitted?

Typhoid fever is a generalized disease caused by the typhoid bacillus. It is transmitted from infected food, milk, or water (usually contaminated by sewage). It can be spread by flies but also by direct contact with infected material.

What is a "typhoid carrier"?

This is a "healthy" person who had typhoid fever at one time, who recovered from it, but still harbors the live germs in his body. He can act as a source of widespread contamination in a community, especially if he has anything to do with the handling of food.

What are the methods of preventing the spread of typhoid fever?

Purification of water supplies and pasteurization of milk are essential measures. Typhoid carriers, when discovered, must be prevented from handling food which is to be used by other people. Typhoid fever must be recognized early and the patient must be isolated from healthy people. All of the typhoid patient's belongings and all of his excretions must be sterilized and kept from contact with other people.

Is vaccination against typhoid fever effective?

Yes. Typhoid vaccine should be taken under the following circumstances:

a. When traveling in a country where the water purity is doubtful and where the disease is known to exist.
b. During typhoid epidemics.
c. When there has been contact with a patient who has the disease.

How is a positive diagnosis of typhoid fever made?

There is a special blood test which becomes positive during the second week of the disease. This is called the Widal test. Also, the germ can be grown in the laboratory from the patient's blood, urine, or stool.

How common is typhoid fever in the United States today?

With the establishment of pure water supplies, the proper handling of food supplies, and the proper isolation of the occasional case, this disease is now quite a rarity in the United States. Also, the advent of the newer antibiotic drugs can kill the typhoid germs readily and thereby prevent the patient from becoming a spreader of the disease.

What is the incubation period for typhoid fever?

Approximately ten to fourteen days.

How long does it take for the disease to run its course?

Usually, about four to six weeks.

What are "rose spots"?

They are small red spots which appear on the skin, usually on the chest and abdomen, from the seventh to the tenth day of the disease.

Are there any serious complications of typhoid fever?

Yes. Rupture of the intestines and intestinal hemorrhage are the two most serious complications, but they do not occur very often.

How soon can the typhoid patient be allowed out of bed?

He can sit up in bed after his temperature has been normal for one week. He may get out of bed about three or four days later.

How can one tell when the typhoid patient is cured?

When repeated stool examinations and cultures are negative for the typhoid germ. This will insure the fact that the patient is not a typhoid carrier.

What is the present-day treatment for typhoid fever?

a. Bed rest.

b. Medications to maintain proper nutrition.

c. Some of the newer antibiotic drugs have proven to be very effective in bringing about a rather prompt cure.

VIRUS PNEUMONIA
(See Chapter 37, on Lungs.)

MALARIA

What is malaria?

It is an infectious disease caused by one of four different types of parasites. It is transmitted by the bite of an infected mosquito or by the transfusion of blood from a malarial blood donor.

Does malaria occur in the United States?

Yes. There are not too many cases, except in the Southeastern states.

Most cases occur in tropical countries where there are many swamp lands in which the mosquitoes breed readily. It is difficult for people in the United States to comprehend that malaria is still one of the world's greatest health problems—particularly in the tropics.

How is the diagnosis of malaria made?

By the finding of a malarial parasite in the blood cells of the patient. The disease may be suspected whenever there are periodic chills and high fever in a person who has recently been in a malarial area.

Is there a vaccine to prevent malaria?

No.

How can the disease be prevented?

By eliminating or controlling the mosquitoes' breeding places, by the use of adequate mosquito netting and screens in an area of infected mosquitoes, and by placing protective screening around the malarial patient so that he cannot be bitten by a mosquito which will then spread the disease to a healthy individual.

Is there an effective treatment for malaria?

Yes. Most cases respond well to the newer drugs, such as atabrine and chloroquine, which are now used instead of the old stand-by remedy, quinine.

Do malarial attacks tend to recur over a period of years if the disease has not been completely eliminated by treatment?

Yes. Formerly, patients often would have malaria, on and off, for many years.

YELLOW FEVER

What is yellow fever, and how is it transmitted?

It is a disease caused by a filtrable virus and transmitted by the bite of a female mosquito (aedes aegypti) which has previously fed upon the blood of a yellow fever patient.

Is yellow fever ever seen in the United States?

No. The last epidemic occurred in New Orleans in 1905. It is prevalent, however, in Western Africa and in certain parts of South America.

Why is the disease of importance today?

Because of the widespread air travel to areas in which yellow fever is prevalent. Great caution must be taken not to introduce even a single case from an infected area. It is also important that travelers from this country remember to be vaccinated against yellow fever before traveling to infected regions.

DENGUE FEVER

What is dengue fever?

It is one of the tropical fevers, also called breakbone fever, caused by a virus and transmitted by the bite of a mosquito.

Can dengue fever be prevented?

Yes, by controlling or eliminating the mosquito which transmits the disease. DDT must be sprayed over the area of the mosquitoes' breeding places.

Is there a vaccine which will prevent dengue fever?

No.

Does dengue fever occur in the United States?

Occasional cases do occur in the Southeastern states.

RELAPSING FEVER
(Recurrent Fever or Tick Fever)

What is relapsing fever, and how is it transmitted?

It is a disease characterized by bouts of fever, with periods of apparent recovery which are followed by recurring bouts of fever. It is

693

caused by a spirochete germ and is transmitted by the bites of lice or ticks.

Where is relapsing fever found?

The louse-borne type is common in Europe, Africa, and India. The tick-borne type is common in the United States.

Is there a vaccine which will protect against relapsing fever?

No.

INFECTIOUS OR EPIDEMIC JAUNDICE
(*Spirochetal Jaundice or Weil's Disease*)

Is infectious jaundice the same disease as infectious hepatitis?

No. This disease is caused by a spirochete germ and is transmitted by contact with rats, either by eating or drinking food or water which has been contaminated by rat feces or urine, or occasionally by rat bite.

Where is infectious jaundice most commonly found, and who is most apt to develop the condition?

It is most common around wharves, mines, and sewers, because rats are more apt to be found in these places. Miners, sewer workers, and wharf men are therefore more apt to contract the disease.

THE RICKETTSIAL DISEASES

What are the rickettsial diseases, and how are they transmitted?

They are a group of infectious diseases, with fever, caused by Rickettsia, which are germs smaller than bacteria but larger than viruses. They are transmitted to man by the bites of lice, fleas, or mites, or by the attachment of ticks to the skin.

Which diseases are caused by the Rickettsia?

Epidemic typhus fever, Rocky Mountain spotted fever, South American spotted fever, "Q" Fever, Scrub typhus, trench fever, and rick-

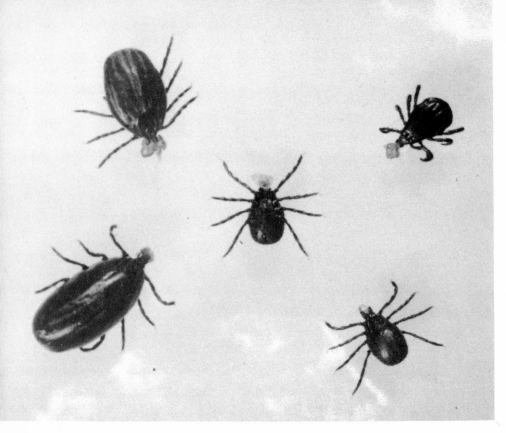

Ticks Which Transmit Tick Fever. Other types of ticks can transmit other diseases, the most serious of which is Rocky Mountain spotted fever. The large size of one tick in the accompanying photograph is caused by the fact that it is gorged with blood that has been sucked from its host. Ticks often double or triple in size after they have fed on blood for a day or two.

ettsialpox. Brill's Disease is a type of typhus fever seen in America, and probably represents a flare-up of a former attack of epidemic typhus fever in a patient who may have had that disease when he lived in Europe, many years prior to the present attack.

How may these diseases be prevented?

By the eradication of fleas, mites, body lice, ticks, and by the control of their breeding places. In tick-infested areas, it is important to inspect the body at frequent intervals to discover any tick attachments to the skin. At night, it is important to use netting to keep insects out.

Are vaccines effective against any of these diseases?

Yes, against typhus fever and Rocky Mountain spotted fever.

Are the rickettsial diseases serious?

Yes, particularly Rocky Mountain spotted fever and certain types of typhus fever, which may lead to death in a rather high percentage of cases if not treated properly.

TULAREMIA
(Rabbit Fever)

What is tularemia, and how is it transmitted?

It is an acute disease caused by a bacillus and characterized by the appearance of a skin sore or ulcer, and it is accompanied by fever which resembles typhoid fever. It is a disease of wild animals, especially rabbits, and is spread among animals by the bites of blood-sucking insects.

How do humans get tularemia?

Most human cases occur in hunters, butchers who skin rabbits or other animals, and farmers and laboratory workers who handle or breed infected rabbits.

How can tularemia be prevented?

By being extremely careful with the handling of wild rabbits and rodents. Care must be exercised in removing ticks from the fur of such animals, and proper clothing must be worn to avoid tick bites. Any wild game that is to be eaten must be very thoroughly cooked.

Is there an effective vaccine against tularemia?

Yes, but to be effective it must be given at least three weeks in advance of possible contact. Hunters, butchers, farmers, and laboratory workers who handle wild rabbits or birds should be inoculated with this vaccine.

What is the treatment of tularemia?

Streptomycin usually cures the disease promptly.

BRUCELLOSIS
(Undulant Fever, Malta Fever, Mediterranean Fever, Gibraltar Fever)

Is brucellosis primarily a disease of humans?

No. It affects animals, usually cattle, swine, and goats. It is caused by a germ called brucella. It is transmitted to man by contact with the secretions and excretions of the above animals and by the drinking of contaminated milk.

Is brucellosis contagious, from man to man?

No.

Who is most apt to contract brucellosis?

It is considered an occupational disease among veterinarians, meat packers, butchers, dairy farmers, and livestock producers.

What are the symptoms of brucellosis?

Fever, chills, body aches and pains, profuse sweating, and loss of weight. The fever is usually intermittent, with long periods of normal temperature. These symptoms may go on for as long as a year or more, and if brucellosis becomes chronic and is untreated, the symptoms may go on for many more years.

Is there an acute form of this disease?

Yes. This lasts only about two to three weeks and must be differentiated from typhoid fever, malaria, or tuberculosis.

How can brucellosis be prevented in man?

By pasteurization of milk. Also, people who handle meat must protect themselves by wearing rubber gloves. All skin lesions should be properly cared for in these people. Infected animals should be detected and destroyed.

What is the treatment for brucellosis?

Streptomycin and sulfa drugs have been found to be most effective. Several vaccines have been used, but they are of questionable value.

697

PLAGUE
(Black Plague, Bubonic Plague)

What is plague?

It is a serious disease which occurred in huge epidemics throughout Europe and Asia in ancient times and in the Middle Ages. It was known as the Black Death. The last great epidemic occurred in India in the early 1900s.

Is plague very common today?

No. There have not been any great epidemics since extensive programs for its extermination have been carried out.

How is the plague transmitted?

The bacteria which cause plague are found in fleas on the bodies of rats. Thus, the fleas from rats get onto the bodies of humans and transmit the disease.

How does one prevent the plague?

By the extermination of rats.

What are the symptoms of plague?

Fever, severe chills, vomiting, great thirst, morning diarrhea, blood spots on the skin, and enlargement of the lymph glands.

What is pneumonic plague?

This is a form of the disease which involves the lungs. It can be transmitted from person to person by droplet infection.

Is plague a serious disease?

Yes. It formerly carried with it a tremendous mortality, but today, with the newer drugs such as streptomycin and the sulfa drugs, the mortality has been reduced from over 90 per cent to less than 20 per cent.

LEPROSY

What causes leprosy?

It is believed to be caused by a germ called Hansen's bacillus.

Is leprosy very contagious?

No. This is a very common misconception. Leprosy is only mildly contagious and its method of transmission is relatively unknown.

Is leprosy found in the United States?

Yes, mostly in the Southern and Gulf states, but the number of cases is small.

What are the symptoms of leprosy?

There may be lumps and thickening of the skin, loss of hair, deformities of bones and joints, and loss of sensation in various areas of the body due to nerve involvement.

What is the outlook in cases of leprosy?

It depends upon the extent and type of involvement. In some cases, after a certain amount of damage has been done, there may be spontaneous disappearance of symptoms, which return at a later date. Other cases go on for twenty years or more.

Is there any effective treatment for leprosy?

Yes. Several sulfone drugs have been used with favorable results. Treatment is carried on in the National Leprosarium, a special government hospital in Louisiana.

INFECTIOUS MONONUCLEOSIS
(*Glandular Fever*)

What is infectious mononucleosis or glandular fever?

It is an infectious disease, probably caused by a virus, which often occurs in mild epidemics among children and young adults, in schools, colleges, and other institutions.

699

How is infectious mononucleosis transmitted?

Probably by air-borne droplet infection.

After exposure, how long does it take for infectious mononucleosis to develop?

Anywhere from five days to two weeks.

What are the main symptoms of infectious mononucleosis?

Fever, headache, generalized aches and pains, and swelling of the lymph glands in the neck, armpits, and groin. The spleen becomes enlarged and certain changes occur in the blood cells. A very prominent symptom at the onset of the disease may be a sore throat.

How can the disease be definitely established?

By certain specific blood examinations.

What is the usual course of infectious mononucleosis?

It is a self-limited disease, with recovery in one to three weeks. The outlook for complete recovery is excellent except in very rare instances. A certain small number of cases may be prolonged for several months.

What are the complications of infectious mononucleosis?

There are not too many, but they may be serious. They include:
a. Throat infection.
b. Liver involvement, with jaundice and hepatitis.
c. Rupture of the spleen.
d. Involvement of the nervous system, with meningitis or encephalitis. This occurs rarely.

What is the specific blood test which clinches the diagnosis of this disease?

The heterophile agglutination test.

Is there any specific treatment for infectious mononucleosis?

No. Antibiotics have been used to prevent secondary bacterial infections, but there is no known cure for the disease itself. Bed rest is very important during the period of fever and for a few days thereafter, and should be prolonged in cases in which liver involvement is suspected. Even though there is no specific treatment, it must be remembered that almost all cases get well by themselves.

Is infectious mononucleosis transmitted by kissing?

It is thought that this occurs, particularly among young adults.

If someone has the type of I.M. (infectious mononucleosis) which persists for several weeks, or even months, must he remain isolated and stay in bed?

No. If his temperature is normal he may be permitted to return to school or work. But such a person should avoid close contact with others, as he may still be capable of transmitting the disease.

RABIES
(*Hydrophobia*)

What is rabies, and how is it transmitted?

It is an acute infectious disease of animals, especially dogs and cats, caused by a virus which affects the nervous system. The virus is present in the saliva of infected animals and is transmitted by the bite of the animal to another animal or to a human.

What is the incubation period of rabies?

Usually, about two weeks, but prolonged periods up to two years following an animal bite have been recorded in rare instances.

What are the symptoms of rabies?

Fever, restlessness, and depression. The restlessness leads to uncontrollable excitement and convulsions. There is excessive salivation, and painful spasms of the throat muscles. Death occurs in three to five days. Because of the spasms of throat muscles, there is fear of drinking or swallowing, thus the term "hydrophobia."

701

What should be done to a dog or other animal which bites a human being?

It should be kept under observation for about two weeks. If it does not become ill or die in this period of time, its bite may be considered harmless and the animal can be released to its owners. If the animal becomes ill, it should not be killed but allowed to die naturally, since this will make the diagnosis easier. An autopsy should then be performed and the animal's brain examined in order to obtain positive proof that the animal had rabies.

Can rabies be prevented and controlled?

Yes, by the impounding and destruction of stray dogs and cats, and by the mass inoculation of licensed dogs and cats against rabies.

What is the treatment for a dog or cat bite?

Thorough washing with soap and water for a period of five to ten minutes is sufficient. Cauterization is no longer considered to be good treatment.

Is there an effective vaccine against rabies and when should it be used?

Yes. Anti-rabies vaccine is very effective in preventing the disease, but it must be used cautiously, as it sometimes has toxic effects. When the animal which caused the bite is known to have the disease or cannot be examined because it cannot be located, immediate vaccination against rabies should be begun. In cases in which the dog is thought to be healthy and can be observed, the animal should be watched for fourteen days. If the animal remains healthy, it is not necessary to vaccinate the human. If the dog becomes ill and dies, immunization of the bitten person should be started at once.

Can rabies be prevented if one waits several days after the bite before starting the vaccination?

Yes. It is safe to wait and see what happens to the animal before starting to give rabies vaccination.

If a human being once develops rabies, what is the outcome?

Rabies is fatal in almost 100 per cent of cases and there is no known treatment of any value.

TETANUS
(*Lockjaw*)

What is tetanus, and what causes it?

It is an acute infectious disease causing spasm of muscles and convulsions. The spasm of the jaw muscles accounts for the name "lockjaw." The disease is caused by a bacillus which can survive in extreme heat or cold for many years because it forms inert "spores" which may become activated after they enter the body of a human.

How is tetanus transmitted?

The germ is distributed widely throughout the world, especially in soil which has been contaminated or fertilized by animal or human feces. Wounds, especially deep puncture wounds which are contaminated, form excellent sites for the development of tetanus. The germ forms a toxin which acts upon nerves in the brain and spinal cord and leads to muscular spasms and convulsions.

What is the incubation period of tetanus?

Between five and ten days, but it may vary from two days to two months.

How is the diagnosis of tetanus made?

A history of recent injury or operation is given. The wound appears infected, and upon taking cultures of the pus, the tetanus germ is found. The symptoms must be distinguished from those of meningitis, rabies, or other conditions.

How can tetanus be prevented?

By the use of:

a. Tetanus toxoid—for active immunization of people liable to injuries, such as gardeners, farmers, soldiers, mechanics, children,

703

athletes. This produces prolonged immunity that must be continued by a yearly booster injection.

b. Tetanus antitoxin (TAT)—for passive immunization. Once an injury has occurred, this will afford protection of short duration.

What is the outlook once tetanus has developed?

It depends upon the promptness with which treatment is begun. The mortality rate is very high, especially in the very young and very old. The mortality rate varies from 30 to 100 per cent. If the patient survives the first nine or ten days, his chances for full recovery are considered improved.

What is the treatment for tetanus?

a. Huge doses of antibiotics.

b. The giving of large doses of tetanus antitoxin.

ANTHRAX

What is anthrax, and how is it transmitted?

It is a highly infectious disease of animals which is caused by the anthrax bacillus and can be transmitted to man directly or indirectly. It occurs chiefly in goats, cattle, sheep, horses, and hogs. Thus, people who have contact with these animals are prone to develop the disease.

How do humans develop anthrax?

The germs usually enter the skin through a small cut or laceration on the hands of people who habitually handle the animals mentioned above. Also, by breathing in anthrax germs, the lungs may become infected. Or if infected material from the animals is swallowed, intestinal involvement may develop.

What is the treatment for anthrax?

Antiseptic dressings and antibiotics should be applied to local wounds, and anti-anthrax serum should be given in large doses.

What is the outlook once anthrax has developed?

Four out of five people will recover, if properly treated.

Is anthrax common?

Not any more, because people who handle animals that have anthrax sores are now fully aware of the possibility of catching the infection. Such people now take proper precautions.

ECHO VIRUS DISEASE

What is ECHO Virus Disease?

It is a contagious viral infection affecting the intestinal, respiratory and nervous systems; seen most often in young children but also occasionally in adults. Frequently, it occurs in large epidemics.

What are the symptoms and course of ECHO Virus Disease?

Fever, headache, pain and stiffness in the neck and back, vomiting, sore throat, abdominal cramps and diarrhea. The usual course is spontaneous, complete recovery within 3 to 5 days.

Are specific medications necessary to cure ECHO Virus Disease?

No. Usually, aspirin for the aches and pains, and drugs to relieve the vomiting and diarrhea are sufficient. Antibiotics are not indicated.

Is ECHO Virus Disease serious?

No, but it is sometimes erroneously diagnosed as polio or meningitis, thus alarming the family.

32 Inherited and Congenital Conditions

What is meant by an inherited characteristic?

It is a trait or bodily characteristic which is passed on from one generation to another. Such a trait or characteristic is determined by units within the nucleus of the germ cells, called chromosomes or genes.

What is meant by a congenital condition?

A trait or bodily characteristic with which one is born, usually as a result of something which happens to the embryo during its development or at birth. For example, if the mother develops German measles during the early weeks of pregnancy, this is likely to affect the growing embryo and produce blindness, heart disease, and other conditions. Under such circumstances, these conditions would be regarded as congenital, since they occurred during the formation of the embryo and were *not* inherited.

Do inherited characteristics tend to follow any pattern of inheritance?

Yes. The Mendelian law governs inheritance.

What is the difference between a dominant and a recessive characteristic?

A dominant characteristic is much more likely to appear in the off-

BROWN EYES

PARENTS:
One pure Brown eyes
and one pure Blue eyes

BLUE EYES

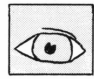

CHILDREN:
Eyes Brown (dominant) with Blue recessive

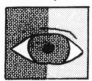

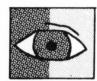

PARENTS:
with Brown dominant and Blue recessive

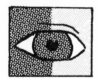

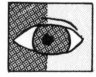

CHILDREN:

| ¼ will be pure Brown | ½ will be Brown dominant and Blue recessive | ¼ will be pure Blue |

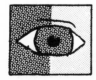
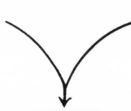
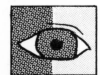
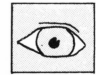

Mendelian Law. The above illustration is a schematic representation of the Mendelian Law as it applies to the inheritance of eye color. The same law applies to inheritance of other physical characteristics.

spring than a recessive one. For instance, with one brown-eyed and one blue-eyed parent, the chances are that more of the children will be brown-eyed, as brown eyes is the dominant characteristic. When a child has parents with black hair but is born with red hair, red hair is the recessive characteristic.

Are most inherited defects and deformities dominant or recessive characteristics?

Most of them are recessive characteristics and will appear in only a small percentage of cases.

Do inherited characteristics sometimes skip generations and appear in subsequent generations?

Yes.

If someone has an inherited deformity, is there a tendency for his children to have this deformity?

Yes, but it must be remembered that inherited defects occur in only a small percentage of offspring. However, a family with known inherited defects has a much greater chance of having children with these defects than does a family in which there are no known inherited abnormalities.

Is it safe for two people, each of whom has a family history of inherited deformities, to marry one another?

Yes, but they must carefully consider the possibility of passing on an abnormality to their children. It is wise for such a couple to seek expert advice before having children.

Is it safe to marry a relative?

It is safe to marry a relative but it is wise not to have children when the relationship is close. This is apt to bring out undesirable recessive traits.

Is it safe to marry into a family in which there is known insanity?

Yes. Insanity is not inherited, although the tendency to inherit personality disorders may occur in some families. Environmental factors are usually much more important.

What are some of the common inherited traits and abnormalities?

Color blindness, skin color, eye color, hair color, harelip, clubfoot, cleft palate, twinning or other multiple birth tendencies, body build, mental deficiency, hemophilia, etc. Also, certain allergies and tendencies toward development of other diseases may be inherited.

Is cancer inherited?

No, although the tendency toward the development of tumors might be inherited.

Can paternity be determined accurately?

Yes. By means of certain blood studies, it can be determined with a fair degree of accuracy.

Can events in the life of a pregnant woman alter the physical development of the unborn child?

Illness in the mother may produce a defect in the development of her embryo. This will appear as a congenital abnormality. Emotional upsets which affect the mother during her pregnancy will *not* influence the child.

Can x-ray radiation or exposure to radioactive substances alter the characteristics of offspring or produce abnormalities?

Excessive exposure to x-rays or radioactive substances during the early weeks of pregnancy might influence and disturb the normal development of the embryo. Also, it is now thought that excessive x-ray radiation in the region of the ovaries may cause alteration of some of the cells so that an abnormality might crop up in a child or grandchild. This entire subject is now undergoing very intensive investigation.

Is it possible to avoid having children who will inherit abnormalities from their parents?

This question is related to the general problem of preventive medicine in relation to hereditary disease. First, it might be well to avoid mating with a family known to have inherited diseases. Second, relatives who marry one another should seriously consider the inadvisability of having children. This relationship, called consanguinity, may bring out undesirable latent hereditary taints.

Are intellect and intelligence inherited?

It is difficult to assess the relative role of heredity and environment in this connection. It is known, however, that intelligent people have a greater tendency to have intelligent children. How much of this is due to their environment we cannot now state. It is known that mental retardation is often inherited or may result from a birth injury or infection.

Should people who have one abnormal child risk having other children?

Many abnormalities are now known to be the result of conditions which occurred during pregnancy or at birth, and therefore would not affect subsequent children. Of the inherited conditions, many are recessive and the chance of other children being affected is small. Expert medical advice is available and should be sought in such cases.

Should people with inherited defects marry and have children?

They may marry, but they should carefully consider whether they ought to have children, and the advice of medical experts should be obtained. Some inherited conditions are recessive and will affect only a few scattered members in a family tree. Other inherited disorders run a dominant pattern and the chances of their appearance in the children are great. In such cases, it might be wiser for a couple to adopt a child rather than have their own.

Should people who have had defects such as clubfoot or harelip, etc., exercise more than the usual care in the selection of a mate?

Yes. They ought to avoid mating with anyone with similar family history or defects.

Is longevity inherited?

No, but the tendency toward longevity may be inherited. (See Chapter 5, on Aging.)

Should one exercise caution in marrying into a family in which there are several members who have had epilepsy or mental disorders?

Yes.

Are weight and height characteristics inherited?

Height is much more likely to be inherited than weight. Weight will depend upon one's eating habits, which are usually environmental in nature and not inherited. However, a tendency toward obesity may exist in certain families.

Is it serious if a pregnant woman develops German measles?

Yes. If it occurs during the first few months of pregnancy, it may lead to blindness, deafness, or heart disease in the offspring.

Are personality traits inherited?

Heredity may play a role in the development of personality, but it is probably a small one. The most important contribution to personality development is the environment in which the child grows up.

Is there any truth to the statement that a "black sheep" is one who has inherited certain unfavorable characteristics from an ancestor?

No.

Are criminal tendencies inherited?

No.

Is there any such thing as inheriting a "weak character"?

No.

Are many diseases inherited?

No. Your physician will be able to inform you precisely as to which diseases are inherited. They are relatively few in number.

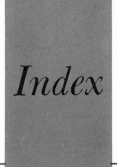 *Index*

This Index lists the entries for this particular volume only. For a complete Index listing all entries in the entire four volumes of this New Illustrated Medical Encyclopedia, *see back of Volume Four.*

ABDOMEN
    acute, and ovarian cysts, 504
    fluid accumulation, 502, 504, 570
    pain, 466, 472, 479, 488, 492, 499, 511
        colicky, 522, 555-556, 679-680, 686
        in ECHO virus disease, 705
    peritonitis, 488, 491
    pressure from coughing, 600
Abdominal organs. *See* specific organs
Abnormalities, birth. *See* Congenital defects
Abortion, 481-495
    complete, 481, 482, 483
    criminal or illegal, 466, 481, 484-486
    and curettage, 483, 484
    and endometritis, 466-467
    and fibroid, 474
    habitual, 484
    hospitalization need, 484, 485-486
    incomplete, 467, 481, 483, 484
    induced, 481
    inevitable, 481, 482, 483
    and infection, 483, 484-485
    missed, 481, 483-484
    resumption of activities after, 485
    spontaneous, 481, 482
    sterility after, 485, 486
    and syphilis, 450
    therapeutic, 481
        legal indications, 485
    threatened, 481, 482-483
    "tubal," 492
Abrasion
    corneal, 402-404
    first-aid treatment, 402, 538-540
        foreign bodies, 402, 524

Abscesses
    See also Infections
    Bartholin, 435-436, 449
    brain, 364, 366
    drainage, 435-436
    and ear infections, 361, 364, 366
    Fallopian tubes, 488-489
    of ovary, 477, 488
    and sepsis of newborn, 653-654
    teeth, and earache, 362
Achalasia, 382, 387, 388-389
Acid, burns due to, 516
Accidents. *See* First-aid treatment
Acidity
    stomach, 384, 556
    vaginal, 446
Acoustic nerve, 359, 363, 370, 375, 376
    See also Ear
Adenoids, and otitis media, 362, 364
Adhesions
    and endometrial implants, 479
    Fallopian tubes, 479, 491
    for retina reattachment, 419
    valvular, 595
Age. *See* Aging; Child; Infant; Puberty
Aging
    and cancer, 455, 469-470
    and coronary artery disease, 584
    and endometrial hyperplasia, 468-469
    and gall bladder, 550
    and hernias, medical management, 603
    and hysterectomy, 469, 477
    and longevity, 710
    and menopause. *See* Menopause
    and senile vaginitis, 446, 447